# FIRST AID FOR THE
# NEUROLOGY
# CLERKSHIP

# NOTICE

Medicine is an ever-changing science. As new research and clinical experience broaden our knowledge, changes in treatment and drug therapy are required. The authors and the publisher of this work have checked with sources believed to be reliable in their efforts to provide information that is complete and generally in accord with the standards accepted at the time of publication. However, in view of the possibility of human error or changes in medical sciences, neither the authors nor the publisher nor any other party who has been involved in the preparation or publication of this work warrants that the information contained herein is in every respect accurate or complete, and they disclaim all responsibility for any errors or omissions or for the results obtained from use of the information contained in this work. Readers are encouraged to confirm the information contained herein with other sources. For example and in particular, readers are advised to check the product information sheet included in the package of each drug they plan to administer to be certain that the information contained in this work is accurate and that changes have not been made in the recommended dose or in the contraindications for administration. This recommendation is of particular importance in connection with new or infrequently used drugs.

# FIRST AID FOR THE
# NEUROLOGY CLERKSHIP

**Michael S. Rafii, MD, PhD**
*Medical Director*
*Alzheimer's Therapeutic Research Institute (ATRI)*
*Professor of Neurology*
*Keck School of Medicine*
*University of Southern California*
*Los Angeles, California*

New York   Chicago   San Francisco   Lisbon   London   Madrid   Mexico City
New Delhi   San Juan   Seoul   Singapore   Sydney   Toronto

*First Aid for the Neurology Clerkship*

1 2 3 4 5 6 7 8 9   DSS   28 27 26 25 24 23

**ISBN 978-1-264-27884-8**
**MHID 1-264-27884-5**

This book was set in Minion Pro  by MPS Limited.
The editors were Bob Boehringer and Christie Naglieri.
The production supervisor was Catherine Saggese.
Project management was provided by Alok Singh, MPS Limited.

This book is printed on acid-free paper.

**Library of Congress Cataloging-in-Publication Data**

Names: Rafii, Michael S., editor.
Title: First aid for the neurology clerkship / editor, Michael S. Rafii.
Description: New York : McGraw Hill, [2023] | Includes bibliographical
   references and index. | Summary: "First Aid for the Neurology Clerkship
   is a high yield, clinically relevant resource covering all important
   topics and principles needed to succeed in the neurology clerkship and
   shelf examination. The content organization is mirrored directly after
   standard clerkship objectives and the Neurology shelf exam blueprint. It
   focuses on clinical scenarios and provide details to help the reader
   understand the disease process and how to differentiate the process from
   other disorders. The pharmacology content focuses on medications
   specifically targeting neurologic diagnoses, as well as recreational or
   street drugs. Overall, it gives students a high yield content foundation
   for everything they will be expected to know"—Provided by publisher.
Identifiers: LCCN 2022038586 | ISBN 9781264278848 (paperback ; alk. paper)
   | ISBN 1264278845 (paperback ; alk. paper) | ISBN 9781264278855 (ebook)
Subjects: MESH: Nervous System Diseases | Clinical Clerkship |
   Neurology—education | Outline
Classification: LCC R839 | NLM WL 18.2 | DDC 610.71/1—dc23/eng/20230206
LC record available at https://lccn.loc.gov/2022038586

# DEDICATION

To the contributors to this and future editions, who took time to share their knowledge, insight, and experience for the benefit of medical students.

And

To the patients who inspire, motivate, and teach us every day and night.

And

To our families, friends, and loved ones, who endured in the task of assembling this guide.

# CONTENTS

# CONTRIBUTING AUTHORS

**ASHIM AHUJA, MD**
*Resident in Neurology*
*Keck School of Medicine*
*University of Southern California*
*Los Angeles, California*

**JEFFREY GOLD, MD, PhD**
*Clinical Professor of Neurology*
*University of California, San Diego*
*La Jolla, California*

**DANIEL GUILLEN, MD**
*Assistant Professor of Neurology*
*University of Tennessee Health Sciences Center*
*Memphis, Tennessee*

**JENNIFER S. HUI, MD**
*Neurology Residency Program Director*
*Associate Professor of Neurology*
*Keck School of Medicine*
*University of Southern California*
*Los Angeles, California*

**ABHI H. KAPURIA, MD**
*Neurologist*
*Telespecialists Teleneurology*
*Durham, North Carolina*

**ARIEL LEFLAND, MD**
*Neuroimmunology Fellow*
*Yale University School of Medicine*
*New Haven, Connecticut*

**DANIEL M. OH, MD**
*Vascular Neurology Fellow*
*Keck School of Medicine*
*University of Southern California*
*Los Angeles, California*

**SANDHYA RAVIKUMAR, MD**
*Neurology Clerkship Director*
*Assistant Professor of Neurology*
*Keck School of Medicine*
*University of Southern California*
*Los Angeles, California*

**VINOD RAVIKUMAR, MD**
*Assistant Professor of Neurology*
*New York Medical College*
*Valhalla, New York*

**MISHY ROY, MD, MHA**
*Chief Resident in Neurology*
*Duke University Medical Center*
*Durham, North Carolina*

**HANS H. SHUHAIBER, MD**
*Assistant Professor of Neurology*
*University of Florida*
*Gainesville, Florida*

**SARAH WIEGAND, DO, MSc**
*Assistant Professor of Neurosciences*
*University of California San Diego*
*San Diego, California*

# CONTRIBUTING AUTHORS

# REVIEWERS

**YUSUF MEHKRI, BS**
*Medical Student*
*University of Florida College of Medicine*
*Gainesville, Florida*

**CHELSIE ANDERSON, MD, MS**
*Resident in Surgery*
*University of California, San Francisco*
*San Francisco, California*

**BENJAMIN STUART, MD**
*Neurocritical Care Fellow*
*University of Southern California*
*Keck School of Medicine*
*Los Angeles, California*

**SEAN BLITZSTEIN, MD**
*Clinical Professor of Psychiatry*
*University of Illinois, Chicago*
*Chicago, Illinois*

# PREFACE

With *First Aid for the Neurology Clerkship,* we hope to provide medical students with the most useful and up-to-date preparation guide for the Neurology Clerkship. This book represents an outstanding effort by a talented group of authors and includes the following:

- A practical guide on how to succeed in the neurology rotation
- Real-world advice on test-taking and study strategies
- Concise summaries of hundreds of testable topics
- High-yield tables, diagrams, and illustrations
- Key Facts and Wards Tips in the margins highlighting "must know" information
- Mnemonics throughout, making learning memorable and fun

We invite you to share your thoughts and ideas to help us improve *First Aid for the Neurology Clerkship;* Kindly reach out at FAneuroclerkship@gmail.com

San Diego, Michael S. Rafii

# ACKNOWLEDGMENTS

This study guide has been a collaborative project from the start. We gratefully acknowledge the thoughtful comments and advice of medical students, residents, and faculty who have supported the authors in the development of *First Aid for the Neurology Clerkship*.

Thanks to the publisher, McGraw Hill, for supporting this effort. For his enthusiasm, support, and commitment to this project, thank you to our editor, Bob Boehringer. A special thanks to Christie Naglieri for her remarkable production work.

# CHAPTER 1

# INTRODUCTION

In this chapter, we will provide an overview of the typical neurology clerkship. We focus on its goals and provide tips on how to succeed in the clinic, on the wards, and on the shelf exam (eg, National Board of Medical Examiners). Most medical schools now require a 4- or 6-week rotation that introduces students to the vast, and sometimes intimidating specialty of neurology. Often, there is both an outpatient and inpatient experience as well as exposure to some of the subspecialities within neurology such as stroke, movement disorders, neuro-critical care, and epilepsy.

## Why Do the Neurology Clerkship?

- The brain and nervous system are fascinating!
- There is an explosion in new diagnostics and therapeutics.
- Regardless of which branch of medicine you specialize in, you will encounter patients with neurological disease.
- Neurological diseases affect a large and increasing population globally.
- The pathophysiology of neurological disorders is extremely diverse.
- There are many opportunities for research and academic careers.
- All practice settings are possible and in high demand:
  - Private practice (inpatient and/or outpatient)
  - Managed care groups
  - Academic practice—research/education
  - Hospitalist positions (inpatient only)
  - Telemedicine
  - Locum tenens
  - Part-time or full-time

## Components of the Neurology Clerkship

- Most neurology rotations include time in outpatient neurology clinics and/or inpatient neurology or consult services.
- Some important neurological diagnoses that you will encounter and should become familiar with include:
  - Stroke
  - Headache
  - Seizure
  - Dementia
  - Multiple sclerosis
  - Parkinson's disease
  - Peripheral neuropathy
  - Myasthenia gravis
  - Amyotrophic lateral sclerosis

## How to Succeed in the Neurology Clerkship

- Maintain a positive and teachable attitude.
  - Even if neurology is not for you, your goal is to learn some of the important aspects of neurology. If you are enthusiastic and eager to learn, then your team will be more excited to teach and involve you in patient care.

- Be well prepared, starting from Day 1.
  - Here is a suggested list of neurological exam tools.
    - Penlight
    - Visual acuity cards
    - Tongue depressor
    - Tuning forks (128 Hz and 256 Hz)
    - Weighted reflex hammer
    - Safety pins
    - Ophthalmoscope (optional)
- Familiarize yourself with the neurological examination.
  - Repetition is the best way to learn. Practice the neuro exam on friends and family members. If you practice doing enough neurological exams that are normal, then it is easier to identify abnormalities when they occur.
  - Use the same order every time so that it is easier to keep track of every part of the exam.
  - Make sure you give yourself enough time in the morning to obtain sign-out from the overnight team, chart review your patients, examine your patients, discuss the case with your team, and make it to rounds on time.
- Be a team player.
  - Anticipate what your neurology team needs.
    - Volunteer to see new patients.
    - Assist with communication with consultants, primary teams, or other members of the healthcare team (nurses, physical therapists, occupational therapists, social workers, case managers).
    - Keep your patients and their families updated.
    - Help assist with procedures such as lumbar punctures.
  - Support your fellow medical students and help each other out when needed. Developing camaraderie is an essential part of training, as the most successful residents are those who can easily work with their colleagues.
- Take ownership of your patients.
  - Try to know your patients better than anyone else on the team.
  - Be proactive in obtaining a patient's history and knowing all the relevant details. If your patient is unable to provide history, then this may involve talking to family or caretakers for a more complete story.
  - Follow up on new studies that come back throughout the day and update your team on the newest information.
  - Try to familiarize yourself with barriers to care, or specific disparities that may affect your patient's access to care.
  - In addition to morning rounds, check in on your patients after rounds or before you go home.
  - Try to read your own imaging—this is the best way to learn.
- Time is brain!
  - Work on developing the skill of quickly triaging between "acutely ill" and "not acutely ill."
  - If there is a sudden exam change in your patient, inform your team immediately.

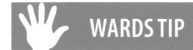

**WARDS TIP**

Pay attention when the attending or residents are doing the neurological exam including the order in which they administer the exam.

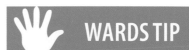

**WARDS TIP**

Practice summarizing a case to its most relevant parts. Try to focus on key findings in the history and exam.

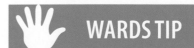

**WARDS TIP**

Whenever possible, review images with the radiologists and try to correlate imaging findings with the patient's history and exam.

- Practice oral presentations and documentation.
  - You will be evaluated on your ability to:
    - Obtain an accurate and comprehensive history.
    - Summarize the neurological exam with any relevant findings.
    - Utilize the SOAP (Subjective/Objective/Assessment/Plan) note format.
    - Formulate an assessment that includes a concise summary, neurological exam synopsis, localization, and differential. The Assessment is the most difficult part of the note to write, but it is also the most important.
  - Oral presentations during rounds can be intimidating at first and become easier with practice. Be concise in your presentation.
- Ask for feedback.
  - Actively ask your team for feedback on your neurological exam, presentations, and notes.
  - Try to immediately implement the feedback that you receive.
- Keep reading.
  - Read about each of your patients' diagnoses.
  - Familiarize yourself with important clinical trials and articles that may be discussed during rounds.
- Maintain professionalism.
  - Be respectful of your patients and their families.
  - Treat the entire healthcare team (ie, attendings, residents, medical students, nurses, and consultants) with respect.
- Maintain confidentiality.
  - Do not discuss patients in the elevator or in public spaces.
  - You may be receiving daily paper patient sign-outs—do not lose or misplace these.

## How to Succeed on the Neurology Exam

- Skim this book before the start of the rotation.
- First two weeks of the rotation: read this entire book while taking notes.
- Two weeks before the exam: review your notes.
- One week before the exam: test your knowledge with practice exams and question banks.
- Three days before the exam: skim this book.
- One day before the exam: skim your notes, exercise, eat well, and get a good night's sleep.
- Read up about cases throughout the rotation and add to your notes.
  - Don't be afraid to ask attending faculty for clarification on study questions.
  - Ask neurology residents lots of questions.
- Study with friends—This is a great way to review material including cases.

- Use different learning modalities.
  - American Academy of Neurology (AAN) Medical Student Educational Resources—access through AAN.com
    - Case study videos
    - Student interest group in neurology (SIGN) webinars
    - Neurology shelf exam review—slide presentations
    - Neurology podcasts

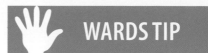

**WARDS TIP**

Review medications, their indications and importantly their side effects.

# NOTES

One of the main goals of the neurology clerkship is to learn how to concisely obtain the patient's history and efficiently perform the neurological examination to arrive at a broad differential diagnosis that can be narrowed down with imaging or laboratory tests. In this chapter, we will cover how to obtain a solid history and perform a comprehensive neurological exam that will help you generate a differential and clinch the diagnosis.

## Obtaining a Neurological History

**Chief complaint:** Make sure to establish the current symptom(s). Clarify the nature of the symptom(s). For example, "dizziness" may mean different things to different patients: lightheadedness, vertigo, unstable gait, confusion, double vision, etc.

**History of present illness:** Interpret symptoms based on chronicity and change over time. Evolution over time and how long it takes for symptoms to present often help identify the etiology. Generate a list of possible causes (differential diagnosis) that will be tested (and confirmed) by your exam, imaging, and laboratory tests. Obtain general history including age, sex, and handedness (90% of the population is right-handed and left hemisphere will be dominant for language; however, in left-handed people, up to 1/3 may have language localized to the right hemisphere).

Sometimes there can be an acute presentation of a chronic disease. Think about the constellation of symptoms that may clue you into an underlying disease, for example, left carotid stenosis can present with recurrent symptoms of slurred speech (dysarthria) and right arm weakness occurring repeatedly over the course of a few weeks (Table 2-1).

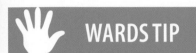

### WARDS TIP

Metabolic derangement can develop over days or weeks but present acutely.

### KEY FACT

If there are concerns about altered mental status or impaired memory, obtain, or confirm, the history with family members.

| TABLE 2-1. Acuteness of Presentation versus Etiology | | | | | | | | | |
|---|---|---|---|---|---|---|---|---|---|
| Acuteness vs Etiology | Vascular | Infectious/ Inflammatory | Trauma | Autoimmune | Migraine | Iatrogenic | Neoplasm | Seizure | Congenital/ Genetic and Degenerative |
| Seconds | Stroke | | TBI | | | | | Generalized or Focal | |
| Minutes | Venous thrombosis | | | | Cluster headache | Sedation with benzo-diazepines | | | |
| Hours | | ADEM | | NMO/MS | Hemiplegic migraine | Dystonia with anti-emetics | | | |
| Days | | Bacterial meningitis | | NMO/MS | | Paresthe-sias with topiramate | | | |
| Weeks | | Myositis | | Anti-NMDA encephalitis | | Seizures with wellbutrin | Glioblas-toma mul-tiforme | | |
| Months | | | | | | Tardive dyskinesia | Acoustic neuroma | | SMA |
| Years | | | | | | | | | Huntington's disease |

ADEM, acute demyelinating encephalomyelitis; MS, multiple sclerosis; NMO, neuromyelitis optica; SMA, spinal muscular atrophy.

**Neurological review of symptoms:** Ask about common neurological symptoms such as dizziness, seizures, headaches, loss of vision, double vision, difficulty speaking, clumsiness, difficulty performing previously known simple tasks, weakness, numbness, abnormal movements, change in behaviors, sleep problems, and confusion/getting lost.

**Past neurological history and relevant medical history:** Include a full past medial history as comorbidities may be important contributors to the current presentation or may be part of an overall syndrome.

**Medication history:** Some drugs can cause neurological symptoms or could be clues to other diseases that the patient could have forgotten to mention. For patients with epilepsy, obtain current and prior antiseizure medications. For acute stroke patients, it is important to know about anti-coagulation.

**Family history:** Make sure to include specific neurological diagnoses but also other possible medical conditions in the family. Some examples include:
- Psychiatric disease or suicide in the family: Huntington's disease.
- Sudden death: channelopathies, including some which cause epilepsy.
- Motor delay: muscular dystrophies.
- Hyperthermia with anesthesia: myopathy.

**Social history:**
- Occupation:
  - Exposures to toxins such as organophosphates in farmers may lead to anticholinergic syndrome.
  - Military service, which may be associated with MS or ALS.
  - Construction workers may bring botulism spores into their homes and expose infants.
- Ethnicity:
  - In Behcet's disease, patients come predominantly from the Mediterranean region.
  - Sickle cell disease is more common in African Americans and is associated with Moya Moya disease and strokes.
- Prior travel:
  - History of living in the Caribbean or South America and HTLV1 infections which can present as gait problems and motor weakness or cysticercosis which can present as recurrent seizures.
  - Swimming in stagnant water could be a risk for infection by Amoebas which can present as headaches.

**Birth and developmental history:** Applicable for pediatric or young adult patients. Birth injury is associated with cerebral palsy, which increases the risk of epilepsy. Metabolic diseases would cause developmental arrest or regression.

**Prior neurological workup:**
- **Imaging:** MRI or CT of the brain or spine have broad utility in neurology. CT is most helpful for vascular and trauma etiologies.

**KEY FACT**

History of diabetes or arrhythmias could be big contributors to neurovascular disease.

**KEY FACT**

Myotonic dystrophy usually includes endocrinological conditions as part of the disease.

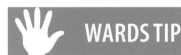

**WARDS TIP**

Anti-cholinergic toxicity inlcudes tachycardia, delirium, hallucinations, mydriasis, dry skin and mucous membranes, urinary retention, decreased gastric motility, and hyperthermia.

**KEY FACT**

Summarize the history with the most relevant information in one or two lines. Formulate a differential diagnosis and then test your hypothesis with the neurological exam.

**WARDS TIP**

In patients with a more acute presentation, such as stroke, time is of the essence. In these situations, you will need to do a rapid assessment, with focused history and targeted neurological exam.

**WARDS TIP**

Consider exam findings that may present as part of an overall condition. Perform a detailed skin exam, including identifying rashes or birth marks.

**KEY FACT**

Some neurological conditions may present as paraneoplastic syndromes, particularly associated with small cell lung cancer, and Pancoast tumor (tumor in the apex of the lung) which could produce a brachial plexitis.

**WARDS TIP**

Thick neck and small palate are risk factors for obstructive sleep apnea, which may underlie headaches, vascular disease, parasomnias, and excessive daytime sleepiness.

- **Electroencephalography (EEG):** To assess for seizures and altered mental status without a clear etiology.
- **Electromyography (EMG):** For peripheral etiologies (muscle, nerve, nerve roots, or anterior horn dysfunction).
- **Cerebrospinal fluid (CSF) studies:** For infections, autoimmune or inflammatory diseases.
- **Other labs:** Chemistries for altered mental status, CBC for systemic infections, genetic testing specific for neurological conditions.

## PHYSICAL EXAMINATION

**General Exam:** Start with vital signs. In cerebrovascular conditions, it is especially important to address blood pressure and heart rate. In neuromuscular diseases, assessing breathing by measuring respiratory rate or oxygen saturation. Pay special attention to irregular heart rhythm or presence of carotid bruits.

## Performing the Neurological Exam

The major components of the neurological exam are:

- Mental status
- Cranial nerves
- Muscle strength, tone, and bulk
- Sensory function
- Coordination
- Reflexes
- Gait

## MENTAL STATUS

Lesions of the brain can result in myriad symptoms. Recognizing the pattern is critical to localizing and generating a differential diagnosis (Table 2-2).

- **Consciousness:**
  - Awake: Patient is interactive and conversational.
  - Drowsy: Decreased level of consciousness, but rapid arousal to verbal or tactile stimuli.
  - Stuporous: Limited arousal to stimuli but continues to have purposeful movements.
  - Comatose: Not arousable.
- **Orientation:** Ask if the patient knows their name, the date (an error of 1-2 days may be acceptable), time of the day, date of birth, and situation.
- **Attention:** Assess by asking the patient to say the months of the year backwards or do series of 7s backwards starting at 100 (this would also address the ability to do calculations). Attention must be tested before

| TABLE 2-2. Localization of Common Mental Status Findings | |
|---|---|
| **Findings** | **Lobe** |
| Apathy, Disinhibition | Frontal |
| Memory issues | Temporal |
| Spatial orientation | Parietal |
| Visual perception | Occipital |

examining short-term memory and inattention. This is one of the key findings in delirium.

- **Memory:** Immediate recall (ask to repeat three unrelated words back to the examiner right after saying them), recent (ask what the patient had for breakfast), remote (the year Neil Armstrong landed on the moon, name the last four presidents).
- **Abstract thinking:** Say a simple, common saying and ask the patient to interpret it, such as "a dime a dozen" or "beating around the bush."
- **Spatial perception:** Assess for ability to copy a drawing, such as an analog clock. Dysfunction is often associated with parietal lobe lesions.

**Dysarthria:** Impaired ability to articulate speech. Voice production requires coordination and normal function of breathing, vocal cords, palate, larynx, tongue, and lips.

- **Spastic:** The patient sounds as if trying to talk from the bottom of the throat. There is abnormal rhythm of the speech. Associated with motor neuron dysfunction in neurodegenerative disease, ie, pseudobulbar palsy or amyotrophic lateral sclerosis (ALS).
- **Extrapyramidal:** It is quiet, breathy, tremorous and nonrhythmic. Seen in Parkinsonism.
- **Cerebellar:** Sounds as if the patient is drunk. Associated with alcohol intoxication, phenytoin toxicity, and hereditary ataxias.
- **Secondary to motor** cranial nerve lesions X, XII, or VII.
  - Nasal: The patient sounds congested.
  - Lingual: Difficulty with t, s, and d sounds.
  - Facial: Difficulty with b, p, m.

**Apraxia:** Inability to perform a motor task.

- **Ideomotor apraxia** localizes to the premotor cortex or dominant parietal lobe. A classic example is dressing apraxia (may ask the patient to unbutton a shirt and button it again).

**Aphasia:** Inability to understand or express speech (Table 2-3).

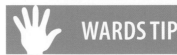

**KEY FACT**

The examiner needs to assess the fluency, comprehension, repetition, naming, reading, and writing.

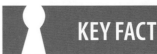

**WARDS TIP**

Ask the patient to repeat "Methodist Episcopal" to test for dysarthria.

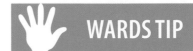

**WARDS TIP**

Myasthenia gravis can present with nasal speech; a key feature is that the speech becomes more nasal as the patient talks more.

**KEY FACT**

Parkinson's disease usually has associated hypophonia, a soft or whisper quality to the voice.

| TABLE 2-3. Types of Aphasias and Associated Findings | | | |
|---|---|---|---|
| **Type** | **Speech Fluency** | **Comprehension** | **Comments** |
| Repetition impaired | | | |
| Broca (expressive) | Nonfluent | Intact | **B**roca = **B**roken **B**oca (*boca* = mouth in Spanish) Broca's area is in inferior frontal gyrus of frontal lobe Patient appears frustrated, insight intact |
| Wernicke (receptive) | Fluent | Impaired | Wernicke's aphasia is **W**ordy but makes no sense Patients do not have insight Wernicke's area is in the superior temporal gyrus of temporal lobe |
| Conduction | Fluent | Intact | Can be caused by damage to ar**C**uate fasciculus. |
| Global | Nonfluent | Impaired | Arcuate fasciculus; Broca and Wernicke areas affected (**all** areas) |
| Repetition intact | | | |
| Transcortical motor | Nonfluent | Intact | Affects frontal lobe around Broca area, but Broca area is spared |
| Transcortical sensory | Fluent | Impaired | Affects temporal lobe around Wernicke area, but Wernicke area is spared |
| Transcortical, mixed | Nonfluent | Impaired | Broca and Wernicke areas and arcuate fasciculus remain intact; surrounding watershed areas affected |

## WARDS TIP

It is important to start observing the patient while obtaining the history.

## WARDS TIP

Be sure to clarify if there is a hearing impairment before starting to evaluate language.

## KEY FACT

Patients with anosmia often report loss of taste in their history.

## WARDS TIP

Olfactory hallucinations, usually of unpleasant odors such as burned rubber, can occur in seizures, especially of the medial temporal lobe (which is usually affected in herpes encephalitis).

## KEY FACT

Papilledema is a sign of increased intracranial pressure and should be concerning for mass lesions, but it is also frequently seen in pseudotumor cerebri. Obtain brain imaging.

## WARDS TIP

Don't perform a lumbar puncture (LP) in the setting of papilledema until brain imaging is done to avoid the risk of causing herniation if there is a mass within the skull.

- **Ideational apraxia** is forgetting how to use an object (may give a pen to the patient and ask to show the examiner how it is used). Usually localizes to the dominant parietal lobe.
- **Speech apraxia** is difficulty generating the movement patterns necessary to produce speech without weakness or difficulty thinking about the words. This may be seen in TBI or stroke affecting the premotor cortex.
- **Oculomotor apraxia** is inability to fully control eye movement. Patients may have difficulty initiating eye movements and may start by turning their heads to compensate. Seen in bifrontal or biparietal hemorrhages as well as in ataxia telangiectasia syndrome.

**Agnosia:** Inability to recognize and identify an object.

**Visual Agnosia:** Unable to see objects properly, unable to copy:
- Due to diffuse brain damage (eg, carbon monoxide) or left occipitotemporal lesion.

**Prosopagnosia:** Inability to recognize faces:
- Due to bilateral PCA infarction.

## CRANIAL NERVES (CN)

*Olfactory Nerve (CN I)*
- Test using a strong smell (ie, coffee), covering one nostril at a time. The most common reason for bilateral anosmia is the blocked passage of both nostrils due to congestion.
- Bilateral anosmia, consider neurodegenerative diseases such as Parkinson's disease, Alzheimer's disease, or Sars-Cov-2 infection.
- Unilateral anosmia is usually blocked nostril versus, very rarely, unilateral frontal masses (meningioma or glioma).

*Optic Nerve (CN II)*
Will involve funduscopic exam, visual acuity, visual fields, and pupils which also involve CN III in its efferent response.
- **Funduscopic exam**

  May use ophthalmoscope or panoptic. Ask the patient to pick a spot far in the opposite side of the room and not to change the focus (it is ok to blink). Many examiners prefer to start with a darker room; however, the pupil will likely constrict regardless due to the light of the ophthalmoscope unless it was chemically dilated. Approach the patient from a 15-degree angle from the side and get closer slowly while adjusting the focus. Assess for the color and margins of the optic disc, characteristics of the blood vessels, and the retina.
- **Visual acuity**

  Evaluate one eye at a time. Test with Snellen chart: Start at 30 cm from the face of the patient and ask them to read from top to bottom; the scoring is on the chart and normal vision should be 20/20.
- **Visual fields**

  Evaluate by confrontation face to face with the patient; cover one eye of the patient and the contralateral eye of the examiner. The examiner and the patient should be looking at each other's eyes. There are two main techniques. The examiner may extend the hand to the periphery and move a finger to the center until the patient is able to see it. The hand of the examiner should be at equal distance from each other, and the patient will

1. Right anopia
2. Bitemporal hemianopia
   (pituitary lesion, chiasm)
3. Left homonymous hemianopia
4. Left upper quadrantanopia
   (right temporal lesion, MCA)
5. Left lower quadrantanopia
   (right parietal lesion, MCA)
6. Left hemianopia with macular sparing
   (PCA infarct)
7. Central scotoma (eg, macular degeneration)

Meyer **L**oop—**L**ower retina; **L**oops around
inferior horn of **L**ateral ventricle.
Dorsal optic radiation—superior retina; takes
shortest path via internal capsule.

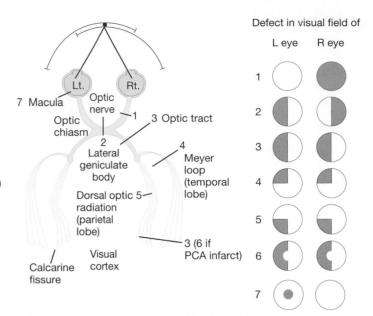

Defect in visual field of

**FIGURE 2-1. Common visual field defects.** From First aid for USMLE Step 1. Reproduced with permission from Bhushan V., Le T., Sochat M., Chavda Y. *First Aid for the USMLE Step 1. 27th ed.* New York: McGraw Hill; 2017.

alert the examiner as soon as they see the fingers. The examiner's visual fields are used as the normal reference. The evaluation is done in four quadrants and then should proceed to the other eye. An alternative is to ask the patient to count fingers in each quadrant. Lesions of the visual pathways can be localized by recognizing the pattern of visual field defect (Fig. 2-1).

■ **Pupillary assessment**

The pupillary response requires an intact CN II (afferent limb) and CN III (efferent limb). Pupillary size varies with intensity of ambient light, but average diameter is 3 to 4 mm. Miosis is less than 2 mm. Mydriasis is over 5 mm.

Anisocoria means pupillary asymmetry. Use the response to light reflex. Start with dim lights. Fix gaze on the opposite wall to eliminate effects of accommodation. Shine a bright light oblique into each pupil. Look for both direct and consensual reaction (contralateral pupil). Record pupil size and shape.

To evaluate for accommodation, lift a finger or a small object about 10 cm from the patient's nose and ask the patient to alternate looking into distance and closer to the patient's nose.

**Possible pupillary findings:**

■ **Anisocoria:** Pupils are unequal but react normally to light.

■ **Holmes Addie pupil:** It presents with anisocoria, results from degeneration of the ciliary ganglia, and is associated with loss of deep tendon reflexes.

■ **Afferent pupillary defect (APD):** Lesion anterior to the optic chiasm. There is no direct or consensual response when flashing the light on the affected side, but both responses are normal when flashing the light in the unaffected side. Seen in Optic Neuritis/Multiple sclerosis.

■ **Efferent pupillary defect:** There is a consensual response but not a direct response when stimulating the affected side with the light. When stimulating the unaffected side, the direct response will be normal but the consensual one will be absent.

## Ocular motility

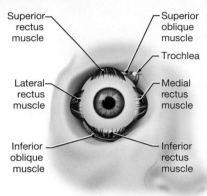

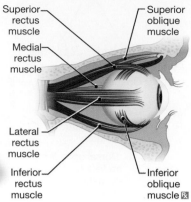

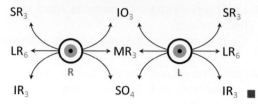

CN **VI** innervates the **L**ateral **R**ectus.
CN **IV** innervates the **S**uperior **O**blique.
CN **III** innervates the **R**est.
The "chemical formula" $LR_6SO_4R_3$.
The superior oblique abducts, intorts, and depresses while adducted.

$SR_3$    $IO_3$    $SR_3$

$LR_6$   MR$_3$   $LR_6$

R    L

$IR_3$    $SO_4$    $IR_3$ ■

**FIGURE 2-2. Innervation of the extraocular muscles.** From First aid for USMLE Step 1. Reproduced with permission from Bhushan V., Le T., Sochat M., Chavda Y. *First Aid for the USMLE Step 1. 27th ed.* New York: McGraw Hill; 2017.

**KEY FACT**

Extreme lateral or vertical gaze may help maximize the diplopia during evaluation. However, if this is chronic, especially congenital, patients do not experience diplopia.

**KEY FACT**

Bilateral CN VI palsy is often a falsely localizing finding that commonly reflects increased intracranial pressure.

- **Argyll-Robertson pupil:** The pupil accommodates to closer objects but does not react to light, usually due to a lesion in the anterior mesencephalon. Most common causes are syphilis and diabetes, and much more rarely, multiple sclerosis (MS).

**Extraocular Movements and Nystagmus (III, IV, VI):** There are four types of eye movements:

- **Saccadic movements:** Rapid movements from one point of fixation to another. Corresponds to the frontal lobe.
- **Persecution movements:** Slow movement that applies to keep gaze fixated on an object that is moving. Corresponds to the occipital lobe.
- **Vestibular positional movement or oculovestibular reflex:** Involuntary movement that compensates for head movement in maintaining fixation. Corresponds to the vestibular nuclei.
- **Convergence movement:** Maintains fixation while objects are getting closer to the face. Only very rarely affected and corresponds to the mesencephalon.

Voluntary eye movements require CN III, CN IV, and CN VI (Fig. 2-2). To test each muscle, ask the patient to move his/her eye following an imaginary H. Initially fixate the head. Then ask the patient to move to a fully adducted position, then up and down, then to a fully abducted position and up and down again. May test for pupillary convergence at the same time. Observe exophthalmos or enophthalmos via the cover/uncover test.

**Common causes of extraocular movement palsies:**

- **Medical:** Diabetes, atherosclerosis, much more rarely vasculitis, CPEO (mitochondrial disease), or Miller Fisher syndrome.
- **Surgical:** Usually when the pupil is affected, consider CN III compression (tumor, aneurysm) or damage (trauma). Anterior communicating artery aneurysm is a common cause of third-nerve palsy.

**Nuclear lesions:** Restricted to the specific nuclei in the brainstem, typically secondary, such as stroke, MS, rarely hemorrhage. Usually associated with other symptoms depending on the localization.

**Lateral gaze palsy** typically corresponds to frontal or parietal lobe lesions.

- In strokes, gaze deviation **falls** toward the side of the lesion.

- In epilepsy, electrical activity **drives** the gaze away from the lesion (seizure focus).
- With lesions in the pons, the patient cannot look toward the paralyzed side.

**Internuclear ophthalmoplegia (INO) also called medial longitudinal fasciculus (MLF) syndrome:** Lesion of the medial longitudinal fascicle, most commonly due to MS and less commonly stroke or pontine glioma. It is a conjugate horizontal gaze palsy. There is a lack of communication such that when CN VI nucleus activates the ipsilateral lateral rectus, contralateral CN III nucleus does not stimulate medial rectus to contract. Abducting eye shows nystagmus. Convergence is normal.

**Horner's syndrome:** Ptosis, anhidrosis, and miosis. It is a lesion of the sympathetic fibers.

**Causes:**
- **Central:** Injury to hypothalamus, brainstem, or superior cervical spine, such as stroke, demyelinating lesions, or more rarely, trauma, or syrinx.
- **Peripheral:** Injury in the sympathetic chain, or in the superior cervical ganglia along the carotid artery. Causes include Pancoast tumor, carcinoma of the bronchial apex, trauma, and less commonly, carotid dissection.

*Nystagmus*
Jerk nystagmus is characterized by direction of the fast phase but caused by a disorder of slow gaze. The slow gaze is the direction toward which the examiner asks the patient to look to, and the fast phase is the rapid beat toward the contralateral direction.

A way to understand the significance of jerk nystagmus: The eyes are slowly "dragged" in an abnormal direction because of vestibular imbalance. They then must "jerk back" to maintain the desired gaze direction.

Examples of nystagmus and localization:
- **Downbeat:** Fast phase downwards. Localizes to the cervicomedullary junction.
- **Rebound:** Horizontal and induced by lateral gaze. Associated with cerebellar dysfunction.
- **Convergence-retraction:** Associated with Parinaud syndrome.
- **Spasmus nutans:** Pendular nystagmus, often asymmetric, episodic, and associated with rapid compensatory head jerk. Usually benign and seen in infants.

*Trigeminal (V) and Facial Nerves (VII)*
For the sensory component of the trigeminal nerve, assess light touch sensation in the forehead, mid face, and lower face. Pinprick may be more precise. The masseter muscle corresponds to the motor function of the trigeminal nerve.

**Facial palsy:** If it is peripheral, including the nucleus, the lesion is ipsilateral, and the forehead is involved (Bell's Palsy). If it is central, the forehead is spared due to input from the upper motor neuron in the cortex to the bilateral CN VII nuclei (Fig. 2-3).

*Vestibulocochlear Nerve (CN VIII)*
Test with finger rubbing at arm's length. If the patient cannot hear strong rubbing, then it is likely impaired.

 **KEY FACT**

Up-gaze palsy is seen in progressive supranuclear palsy (PSP) and in Parinaud syndrome (often due to Pineal gland tumor). The patient may tilt the head back to see straight ahead above the horizon.

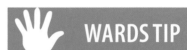 **WARDS TIP**

There is often slight overlap of sensation that crosses the midline of the face. But an exam revealing a perfect midline interruption of sensation would raise concern for a functional neurological disorder.

For the facial nerve, test with lifting eyebrows, eye closure with forceful opening, cheek puff, and smile. Transverse (crooked) smiles or upper lip tenting may reflect bilateral facial weakness.

 **KEY FACT**

Limited facial expression is seen in Parkinsonism, referred to as masked facies.

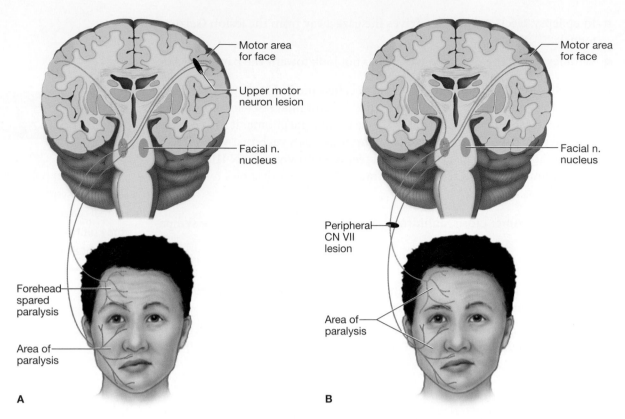

FIGURE 2-3. **Peripheral versus central causes of facial droop.** (**A**) Central CN VII lesion. Crossed fibers allow forehead sparing in an upper motor neuron lesion identifying this presentation as a cerebrovascular accident versus a Bell's palsy. (**B**) Peripheral CN VII nerve lesion causes paresis of both forehead and lower facial muscles. Reproduced with permission, from Knoop KJ, Stack LB, Storrow AB, Thurman R, eds. *The Atlas of Emergency Medicine, 5th ed*. New York, NY: McGraw Hill; 2021.

**Hyperacusis:** May be a sign of stapedial muscle weakness as seen in proximal facial palsy. This is because there is less stability of the ear drum.

**Hearing loss:** The **Weber test** is used to discern between sensorineural versus conductive hearing loss. Place a tuning fork in the middle of the head. Ask the patient on which side it sounds louder.

**Sensorineural hearing loss:** Disease from cochlea to CN VIII. Weber test: Louder in the normal ear.

**Conductive hearing loss:** Disease of tympanic membrane or ossicles → failure to conduct vibration to cochlea. Weber test: Louder in the abnormal ear (Fig. 2-4).

*Glossopharyngeal (IX), Vagus (X), and Hypoglossal (XII) Nerves*
Assess for palate elevation, swallowing, voice, cough, gag. Further details in the description of dysarthria and dysphonia.

Have patient protrude tongue outwards then ask them to push the tongue into the cheek to assess for tongue strength. Note tongue position at rest and on protrusion; the tongue deviates toward the stronger side.

*Spinal Accessory Nerve (CN XI)*
Trapezius muscle strength: Test shoulder shrugs (shoulder elevation). Sterno-cleidomastoid (SCM) strength testing: Place one hand on lower face and have

**KEY FACT**

Slow tongue movements and fasciculations are associated with ALS and fatigability is seen in neuromuscular junction disease such as Myasthenia Gravis.

In patients with prior ENT procedures such as tonsillectomies and adenoidectomies, there may be baseline palate elevation with asymmetry.

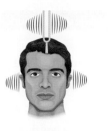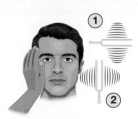

A. Weber test          B. Rinne test

**FIGURE 2-4. Rinne versus Weber test for assessing hearing loss. (A) Weber test:** The vibrating tuning fork is on the midline of the skull. Lateralization of the sound to one ear indicates a conductive loss on that side, or a perceptive loss on the other side. **(B) Rinne test:** The handle of the tuning fork is first placed against the mastoid process then near the external ear. Each time the patient indicates when the sound ceases. Normally, duration of air conduction is twice that of bone conduction. Reproduced with permission from Suneja M, Szot JF, LeBlond RF, Brown DD, eds. *DeGowin's Diagnostic Examination, 11th ed.* New York, NY: McGraw Hill; 2020.

the patient rotate the head toward that side; this activates the contraction of the contralateral SCM.

In functional neurological disease, right shoulder elevation weakness may be seen in association with weakness turning toward the right. This would not follow the physiological distribution of the cranial nerve since the affected accessory nerve should turn the head to the left in this example, away from the weak shoulder elevation.

## MOTOR EXAM

Compare left to right, proximal to distal, arms to legs. Start with observation and look for signs that may represent weakness, such as scapular winging, focal atrophy, scoliosis, or hammer toes.

- **Muscle tone:** Start with passive movement of the extremities.
  - **Hypertonia**
    - **Cogwheeling:** Seen in Parkinsonism or medication side effect from valproic acid.
    - **Spasticity:** Jackknife sensation of the muscle pulling back. It is velocity dependent. Seen in upper motor neuron injury.
  - **Hypotonia**
    - Mainly seen in peripheral nerve and skeletal muscle diseases.
- **Endurance and fatigability:** Can be tested specially with sustained gaze upwards that may lead to ptosis and is a sign of neuromuscular junction disease.

If concern for **psychogenic weakness**, use the **Hoover maneuver**. Ask the patient to lay flat, place one hand under the nonaffected leg and ask the patient to lift the affected side. If there is actual effort, the examiner would feel pressure of the unaffected leg on hand that is placed under the heel; if the weakness is psychogenic, there is no pressure on the contralateral leg. If both legs are affected, test both.

## MUSCLE STRENGTH TESTING

- Direct muscle strength testing is more sensitive to lower motor neuron dysfunction while tests of dexterity and coordination are more sensitive to upper motor neuron dysfunction (Table 2-4).

**KEY FACT**

Do not confuse contractures, which involve a fixed limitation in range of motion, with spasticity. Contractures may be seen in peripheral diseases including Duchenne muscular dystrophy. Contractures do not have the Jackknife (sudden stiffening) component that is seen in spasticity.

| TABLE 2-4. Grading Muscle Strength by the Medical Research Council (MRC) Scale | |
|---|---|
| 0 | No muscle contraction |
| 1 | Visible contraction, but no movement at the joint |
| 2 | Movement at the joint but not against gravity |
| 3 | Movement against gravity but not against resistance |
| 4 | Movement against some resistance but less than full |
| 5 | Movement against full resistance: Normal strength |

## SENSORY EXAM

It is important to explain each test before you do it. The patient's eyes should be closed during testing and the four extremities should be included. Compare side to side and distal to proximal. When you detect any area of sensory loss, map out its boundaries in detail; this is particularly important in pinprick testing. General characteristics include normal, absent, reduced, exaggerated, or perverted (dysesthesias, hyperalgesia).

- **Somatic sensation:** Corresponds to the ascending tracts but does not represent superior function interpretation.
  - **Pain and temperature:** Pinprick testing for pain is preferred. Start distally. If abnormal, try to demarcate an anatomical distribution as this is the best sensation to find dermatomes or specific nerve distributions. Some key findings:
    - Palmar aspect of the index finger corresponds to the median nerve.
    - Palmar aspect of the fifth finger follows the ulnar nerve.
    - Webspace between the thumb and index finger on the dorsal surface of the hand follows the radial nerve.
    - Lateral surface of the foot follows L5.
    - Posterior aspect of the leg follows S1.
    - The web in between the first and second toes follows the peroneal nerve, particularly the superficial peroneal branch.
  - **Light touch/pressure:** Touch lightly randomly, asking the patient if they are feeling the touch.
  - **Vibration:** Use the 256- or 128-Hz tuning fork. First test toe and finger. Ask the patient what they feel, count seconds until the sensation stops, compare side to side; if impaired, test in a more proximal joint.
  - **Proprioception:** Test toes and fingers, move digit only a few degrees, and grab digit from the sides to avoid confusion with pressure sensation. If impaired, move digit greater distance and test more proximally.
- **Interpretive sensation:** Corresponds to cortical function. Typical localization to the parietal lobes.
  - **Stereognosis:** Tested by giving an object to the patient and asking to recognize it; objects often used are pens or coins.
  - **Graphesthesia:** Tested by drawing a number or letter on the palm of the hand and asking the patient if they can recognize it.
  - **Double simultaneous stimulation:** Use light touch, if only one side is felt; this may be a sign of hemineglect, which corresponds to the non-dominant parietal lobe.

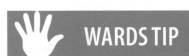

**WARDS TIP**

The examiner can put his/her finger under the finger or toe that is being tested. If you still feel the vibratory sensation, but the patient does not, consider finding as abnormal.

## COORDINATION

Assess control, precision, and synergy of movement. Compare upper and lower extremities and left to right.

To assess tremors, observe at rest and with action. A resting tremor with a pill-rolling motion of the hand is seen in Parkinsonism. On the contrary, essential tremor would be more notable with posture and movement. To elicit them, ask the patient to extend both hands forward with both palms in extension and putting both thumbs very close to each other without touching.

**Archimedes spiral:** Ask the patient to draw a spiral starting in the middle and going into increasingly larger circles. The examiner should draw an initial example. If the patient's spiral is especially small and wavy, consider Parkinsonism; if it has normal size but the waviness gets worse with the outer circles, consider essential tremor.

**Dystonia:** It is an involuntary contraction of muscles resulting in an abnormal posture. In Cervical Dystonia (Torticollis), pressure points are over the obliquus capitis inferior or the splenius capitis muscle, especially when there is a rotation component.

**Maneuvers to test coordination:**

- **Finger-to-nose:** Ask the patient to touch the tip of his/her nose and then the tip to the examiner's finger and go back and forward. Make sure to get full-arm extension. If the patient misses the target, that would be dysmetria, but if the patient's finger wobbles and hits the target, it is more likely ataxia. Tremors may also be observed in this maneuver.
- **Rapid alternating movements:** Ask the patient to tap fingers rapidly, forming an L shape with the index and thumb and then tapping them together, evaluate for speed and rhythm.
- **Heel-to-shin:** With the patient laying down, ask them to put the heel on the contralateral knee and slide down the shin. A common mistake is to test this while sitting, this allows gravity to help the patient.

## REFLEXES AND SPECIAL SIGNS

For deep tendon reflexes, put the muscle in a relaxed position with minimal contraction. Heavier reflex hammers are often more helpful, but you should favor the swing of the wrist instead of a hard hit. It is useful for the examiner to put one finger over the tendon of the muscle being tested to feel the contraction. This allows for localization of the lesion (Tables 2-5 and 2-6).

**The Jendrassik maneuver:** The patient clenches the teeth, flexes both sets of fingers into a hook-like form, and interlocks those sets of fingers together. The maneuver will heighten (exaggerate) lower limb tendon reflexes by countering some of the normal descending inhibition the brain sends to the reflex arc.

| TABLE 2-5. Common Deep Tendon Reflexes and Anatomical Correlations | | |
|---|---|---|
| **Muscle** | **Roots** | **Nerve** |
| Biceps | C5–C6 | Musculocutaneous |
| Triceps | C6–C8 | Radial |
| Patellar | L2–L4 | Femoral |
| Achilles tendon | S1–S2 | Tibial |

**KEY FACT**

Some dystonias are task specific, such as writer's cramp or musician's dystonia; these may require of the patient to perform those tasks in front of the examiner.

**KEY FACT**

In Lambert-Eaton, the reflexes may be absent on initial evaluation, but if there is sustained contraction of the muscle, a reflex may be elicited afterwards.

**KEY FACT**

Reflexes reinforcement: Use isometric contraction of other muscles such as the Jendrassik maneuver, making a fist or teeth clenching when reflexes are difficult to obtain.

| TABLE 2-6. Deep Tendon Reflexes Grading | |
|---|---|
| Absent | 0 |
| Hypoactive | 1 |
| Normal | 2 |
| Hyperactive/Brisk | 3 |
| Markedly brisk, with clonus, contralateral spread | 4 |

## Additional Reflexes and Exam Maneuvers

- **Plantar reflex:** Corresponds to L4-S2, especially S1 and tibial nerve. It is a sign of hyperreflexia or upper motor neuron disease, which is, however, normal in children under 2 years of age. The normal response is a down-going big toe. Abnormal response equals extension and dorsiflexion of the great toe by activation of extensor halluces longus. The most frequently tested is the Babinski reflex by stimulation of the plantar lateral aspect, from the heel toward the fifth and then toward the first digit. Equivalent reflexes include Chaddock (lateral side instead of plantar), Schaeffer (squeezing the Achilles tendon), Oppenheim (pressing knuckles on both sides of the tibial bone), Gordon (squeeze calf muscles), and Bing (light pinprick on the dorsum of the foot).

- **Hoffman reflex:** With the hand relaxed, tap briskly on the top of the nail or the tip of the finger; watch for flexion of the fingers, which is also a sign of hyperreflexia.

- **Jaw jerk:** With complete relaxation of the jaw, type briskly putting a finger on top of the chin and tap briskly on the finger. Feel for a slight jerk. It is usually a sign of neurodegenerative disease or upper motor neuron dysfunction, often seen in ALS.

- **Palmomental reflex:** With both the hand and the face relaxed, scratch slightly in the thenar eminence; may try proximally to distally or distally to proximally monitor for slight contraction of the mentalis muscle. Also, a sign of frontal release as seen in neurodegenerative diseases.

- **Myerson's sign or glabellar sign:** Inability to resist blinking when tapped repetitively on the glabella. May be seen as an early finding in Parkinson's disease and other neurodegenerative diseases.

- **Clinical myotonia:** Defined by limited relaxation of the muscles. By tapping on the thenar eminence, the thumb would go into an adducted position and very slowly relax. There is also limited relaxation after sustained grip, jaw clenching, or blinking.

### MENINGEAL SIGNS

**Meningeal signs:** Neck mobility, look for nuchal rigidity or neck stiffness. Start by asking the patient to lay down flat, then moving the head side to side and then pull up. May also try the Kernig or Brudzinski maneuvers (Fig. 2-5). These signs are often present in the setting of meningitis.

**Kernig's sign:** Severe stiffness of the hamstrings causes an inability to straighten the leg when the hip is flexed to 90 degrees.

**Brudzinski's sign:** Severe neck stiffness causes a patient's hips and knees to flex when the neck is flexed.

---

**KEY FACT**

Consider metabolic derangements, such as hyperkalemia, in the differential diagnosis of patients with muscle weakness and myotonia.

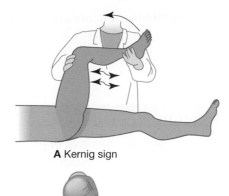

**A** Kernig sign

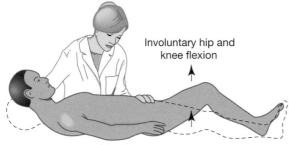

Involuntary hip and
knee flexion

**B** Brudzinski sign

| Physical Exam Finding | Sensitivity (Rule-Out) |
|---|---|
| *Classic Triad Components* | |
| Fever | 85% |
| Neck stiffness | 70% |
| Altered mental status | 67% |
| Absence of all 3 (fever, neck stiffness, AND altered mental status) | 99–100% |
| *Specific Exam Maneuvers* | |
| Kernig sign | 5% |
| Brudzinski sign | 5% |
| Jolt accentuation | 21–97% |

(Greenberg DA, Aminoff MJ, Simon RP. Chapter 1. Neurologic History & Examination. In: Greenberg DA, Aminoff MJ, Simon RP. eds. Clinical Neurology, 8e. New York, NY: McGraw-Hill; 2012.)

**FIGURE 2-5. Testing for meningeal signs.** The Kernig and Brudzinski signs (above); the utility of physical exam findings in ruling out acute meningitis (below). Reproduced with permission from LeBlond RF, DeGowin RL, Brown DD. *DeGowin's Diagnostic Examination. 9th ed.* New York, NY: McGraw-Hill; 2009.

## GAIT

Before assessing gait, make sure that the patient is safe to stand. If the history is concerning for orthostatic hypotension, give some time to transition between sitting and standing. The gait assessment includes the posture, limb movement, length of the steps, speed and rhythm, symmetry, base, steadiness, and turns. Ask the patient to walk regularly, then to walk on toes and heels.

Finally, ask to perform heel to toe walking in a straight line. If unable to perform despite normal strength, consider cerebellar dysfunction, sensory neuropathy, Parkinsonism.

## ROMBERG SIGN

Ability to maintain an upright position with feet together and eyes closed. Start testing with eyes open. Consider it positive if there is a sway or fall when eyes are closed. Indicates impaired proprioception or vestibular dysfunction.

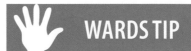

**WARDS TIP**

Nuchal rigidity or stiffness is not observed in infants despite having meningitis.

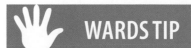

**WARDS TIP**

Patients with a spastic gait may have the tip of one shoe particularly worn out, especially in the lateral aspect of the shoe.

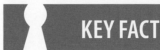

**KEY FACT**

Absence of arm swing when walking could be a sign of Parkinson's disease.

Vision, proprioception, and vestibular function are required for balance control. If either proprioception or vestibular function is compromised, when closing the eyes, relying on only one system would be insufficient, therefore leading to instability or fall.

## Neurological Examination of Unconscious Patients

Patients with altered mental status will not be cooperative following commands; however, a thorough neurological examination can still be obtained.

For **mental status**, evaluate arousal to verbal or tactile stimuli. Noxious stimuli may include sternal rub or nailbed pressure.

**CN II and CN III** may be evaluated by the pupillary reflex or by blinking to light if there is some retention of consciousness.

**CN III, CN IV, and CN VI** can be examined by the oculocephalic reflex (doll's eyes reflex). The patient's eyes are held open, and the head is quickly rotated sideways. The normal response is that both eyes should deviate to the side opposite the direction of head rotation, as if they were maintaining focus on an object. If abnormal, ie, eyes remain fixed straight ahead, it correlates with brainstem dysfunction. Do not perform this reflex on a patient with a C-collar or with concerns for cervical injury.

**CN V and CN VII:** Use the blink reflex. Slightly stimulating the cornea, usually with a wisp of sterile cotton or drop of saline, produces a rapid blink. Avoid stimulating the sclera (whites of the eyes). The afferent stimulation uses the trigeminal nerve (CN V) and the efferent response the facial nerve (CN VII). Other methods include the nasal tickle.

**CN IX and CN X:** Test the gag reflex. The afferent limb of the reflex is supplied by the glossopharyngeal nerve (CN IX). The efferent limb is supplied by the vagus nerve (CN X).

**CN XII:** Assess by observation of the tongue protruding to the midline and looking for fasciculations.

**Reflexes:** They should be obtainable in all four extremities. May be affected by paralytics.

**Motor exam:** Assess for minimal spontaneous movements. May also observe muscle tone and bulk.

**Sensory exam:** If there is some response to tactile stimuli, assess in four extremities to look for asymmetry.

## Interpretation of History and Exam

### LOCALIZATION

The first step is to localize an anatomical area that could explain all the neurological symptoms. Usually, ischemic strokes or MS would follow a clear anatomical distribution, particularly when affecting the cortex. Peripheral injuries that correspond to a specific root or level of the spine would also follow the

| Location of Lesion | Reflexes | Proximal vs Distal | Cranial Nerves | Laterality | Arm vs Leg | Tone |
|---|---|---|---|---|---|---|
| **Cortex** | Increased | — | Contralateral | Unilateral | Usually differently affected | Increased |
| **Basal ganglia** | Increased | — | Contralateral | Unilateral | Symmetrically affected | Increased |
| **Brainstem** | Increased | — | Ipsilateral | Unilateral | Same | Increased |
| **Spinal cord** | Increased | Anatomical level | — | Usually, bilateral | By level | Increased |
| **Anterior horn** | Decreased or absent | Same | — | Variable | Variable | Decreased |
| **Roots, plexus, nerves** | Absent | Anatomical level | — | Unilateral | Per anatomical localization | Decreased |
| **Nerves (GBS)** | Absent | Distal | Bilateral | Bilateral | Legs weaker than arms | Decreased |
| **Junction** | Normal to decreased | Proximal | Motor nerves | Bilateral | Same | Normal |
| **Muscle** | Decreased | Proximal | Motor function | Bilateral | Same | Decreased |

TABLE 2-7. Exam Findings in Patients with a Chief Complaint of Weakness vs Localization in the Nervous System

myotomes or dermatomes. This also applies to focal neuropathies. However, when faced with symptoms that affect both the central and peripheral nervous systems, consider metabolic diseases, vitamin deficiencies, or mitochondrial disease.

Weakness is one of the most common neurological complaints. Table 2-7 helps with localization in patients who present with weakness.

## GENERATING A DIFFERENTIAL DIAGNOSIS

After obtaining the history and performing a neurological exam and localizing the lesion (ie, central or peripheral; brain vs spinal cord; etc.), you can begin to develop the differential diagnosis.

Using VINDICATE mnemonic (V—Vascular, I—Inflammatory/Infectious, N—Neoplastic, D—Degenerative/Deficiency/Drugs, I—Idiopathic/Intoxication/Iatrogenic, C—Congenital, A—Autoimmune/Allergic/Anatomic, T—Traumatic, E—Endocrine/Environment) provides a systematic way to find the type of condition that is affecting the patient.

The combination of etiologies and the localization should narrow down the differential. Once a differential is generated, it may be necessary to ask additional clarifying questions or reassess certain parts of the exam that may be most pertinent before moving on to ordering imaging and laboratory tests.

**Case 1:** A 60-year-old right-handed man presents with a 3-week history of gradually progressive hearing loss of the right ear. He denies vertigo or tinnitus. His ear canals are both clear. There are no associated visual changes. A vibrating tuning fork is applied to the center of his forehead. The sound is louder in his left ear. This finding suggests which of the following?

A. Right ear sensorineural hearing loss
B. Left ear sensorineural hearing loss
C. Right ear conductive hearing loss
D. Bilateral conductive hearing loss
E. Bilateral sensorineural hearing loss

The correct answer is A. The exam is consistent with right ear sensorineural hearing loss. With sensorineural hearing loss, the patient will hear the midline fork more loudly in the unaffected ear. Sensorineural hearing loss is the deafness that develops with injury to the receptor cells in the cochlea or to the cochlear division of the auditory nerve.

**Case 2:** A 35-year-old female with MS presents with blurry vision. Examination reveals that the medial rectus muscle fails to move synchronously with the contralateral lateral rectus muscle on attempted gaze to either side. When each eye is tested individually, medial rectus function is relatively preserved. In addition, prominent nystagmus is present in the abducting eye. These findings indicate evidence of which of the following?

A. Cortical stroke
B. Internuclear ophthalmoplegia
C. Atypical migraine
D. Bilateral vestibular schwannomas
E. Conversion disorder

The correct answer is B. The findings are consistent with MLF syndrome, also called internuclear ophthalmoplegia. Cortical stroke would have additional associated features.

**Case 3:** A 40-year-old man who has received a liver transplant develops fever and headache. When laying supine on the exam bed, severe neck stiffness causes a patient's hips and knees to flex when her neck is flexed. What is the most likely diagnosis?

A. Meningitis
B. Thoracic outlet syndrome
C. Acute herniated disk
D. Sciatica
E. Transverse myelitis

The correct answer is A. The finding is consistent with Kernig's sign, which indicates irritation of the meninges due to bacterial meningitis. Herniated disk and sciatica would include radiating pains. Thoracic outlet syndrome involves the upper extremities. Transverse myelitis would include paresthesia and weakness as well as a sensory level.

# CHAPTER 3

# NEUROANATOMY

In this chapter, we will review neuroanatomical facts that are most likely to show up on the neurology clerkship exam and that you are most likely to be asked about on the wards. In neurology, more than any other disease, structure-function relationships are critical to understanding disease. By keeping a few basic neuro-anatomical rules in mind, you can figure out localization quickly and accurately.

## Central Nervous System

Consists of the brain and the spinal cord, enclosed within the meninges.

### CEREBRUM

The cerebral hemispheres contain areas that have specialized functions (Fig. 3-1). Injury or damage to these areas can result in specific symptoms (Table 3-1).

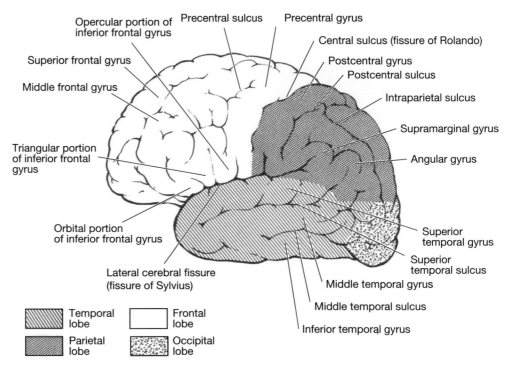

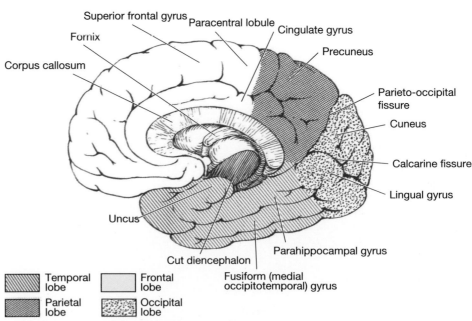

**FIGURE 3-1. Key structures of the cerebral hemispheres.** Reproduced with permission from Waxman SG. *Clinical Neuroanatomy, 29th ed.* McGraw-Hill, 2020.

**TABLE 3-1. Common Brain Lesions Cause Consistent Symptoms**

| Location of Lesion | Consequence | Notes |
|---|---|---|
| Amygdala (bilateral) | Kluver-Bucy syndrome—disinhibited behavior (eg, hyperphagia, hypersexuality, hyperorality) | Associated with HSV-1 encephalitis |
| Frontal lobe | Disinhibition and deficits in concentration, orientation, judgment; may have reemergence of primitive reflexes | Associated with head injury, meningioma or Frontal Demporal Dementia (FTD) |
| Nondominant parietal cortex | Hemispatial neglect syndrome (agnosia of the contralateral side of the world) | |
| Dominant parietal cortex | Agraphia, acalculia, finger agnosia, left-right disorientation | Gerstmann syndrome |
| Reticular activating system (midbrain) | Reduced levels of arousal and wakefulness | Associated with coma |
| Mammillary bodies (bilateral) | Wernicke-Korsakoff syndrome—confusion, ophthalmoplegia, ataxia; memory loss (anterograde and retrograde amnesia), confabulation, personality changes | Associated with thiamine ($B_1$) deficiency and excessive alcohol use, can be precipitated by giving glucose without $B_1$ to a $B_1$-deficient patient. Wernicke problems come in a **CAN** of beer: **C**onfusion, **A**taxia, **N**ystagmus |
| Basal ganglia | May results in tremor at rest, chorea, athetosis | Parkinson's disease, Huntington's disease |
| Cerebellar hemisphere | Intention tremor, limb ataxia, loss of balance: damage to cerebellum → ipsilateral deficits: fall toward side of lesion | Degeneration associated with chronic alcohol use. Cerebellar hemispheres are **lateral**ly located—affect **lateral** limbs |
| Cerebellar vermis | Truncal ataxia, dysartria | Vermis is **central**ly located—affects **central** body |
| Subthalamic nucleus | Contralateral hemiballismus | Can be associated with stroke |
| Hippocampus (bilateral) | Anterograde amnesia—inability to make new memories | Associated with Alzheimer's disease |
| Paramedian pontine reticular formation | Eyes look away from side of lesion | Associated with brainstem stroke |
| Frontal eye fields | Eyes look toward lesion | Associated with stroke or tumor |

Reproduced with permission from T Le, V Bhushan et.al., *First Aid for the USMLE Step 1, 27th ed.* McGraw Hill, 2017.

- Frontal Lobe—extends from the frontal pole to the central sulcus and the lateral fissure
- Parietal Lobe—extends from the central sulcus to the parieto-occipital fissure
- Occipital Lobe—the exterior pole
- Temporal Lobe—below the lateral cerebral fissure and extends back to the level of the parieto-occipital fissure on the medial surface of each hemisphere

## CEREBELLUM

- Involved in body equilibrium and the planning, initiation, and coordination of movement.
- Divided into specific regions (Fig. 3-2).
- Information flows to and from the brain and spinal cord via the cerebellar peduncles, which sit adjacent to the brainstem.
- Unlike cerebral hemispheres, cerebellar hemispheres control the ipsilateral side of the body.

## KEY FACT

Strokes of the cerebellum lead to dizziness, nausea/vomiting, ataxia (patient reports feeling drunk) with falling to affected side. Nystagmus is often absent in these central lesions.

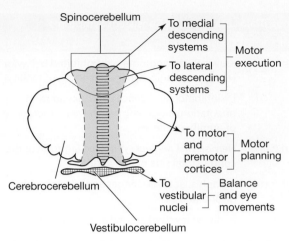

**FIGURE 3-2. Functional anatomy of the cerebellum.** Reproduced with permission from WF Ganong. *Review of Medical Physiology, 22nd ed.* New York. McGraw-Hill, 2005.

The ataxia seen in Wernicke encephalopathy is due to acidosis of the vermis. Excessive and chronic alcohol consumption is associated with thiamine (vitamin B1) deficiency. Thiamine is essential for proper glucose metabolism. Without it, glucose is metabolized through less efficient anaerobic pathways, leading to acidosis. Treatment: High-dose parenteral thiamine must be given prior to refeeding or IV glucose to prevent exacerbation of abnormal glucose metabolism.

## BRAINSTEM

- The three levels of the brainstem from superior to inferior are the midbrain, pons, and medulla.
- Has sensory information coming in and motor information going out for the head and neck.
- Receives vestibular, auditory, taste, and visceral sensory information.
- Motor functions include control of ocular, pupillary, facial, laryngeal, pharyngeal, and visceral musculature.
- The 12 cranial nerves can be divided into three groups of four that mostly correspond to the three brainstem levels with a few exceptions as noted below:
  - Midbrain: 1-2-3-4
  - Pons: 5-6-7-8
  - Medulla: 9-10-11-12

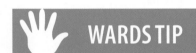

## WARDS TIP

Unilateral lesions of the brainstem cause ipsilateral sensory and/or motor symptoms in the face, but contralateral symptoms in the body ("crossed signs").

## KEY FACT

In Locked-in syndrome, the patient is awake and conscious, but cannot move or communicate with the exception of blinking and vertical gaze. Caused by ventral pontine lesions (eg, basilar artery thrombosis, pontine hemorrhage, or central pontine myelinolysis).

CN 1 and CN 11 do not connect directly to the brainstem.

CN 5 has nuclei at all three levels of the brainstem.

CN 8, the vestibular nuclei are in the medulla and the cochlear nuclei are at the pontomedullary junction.

A number of reflexes can be tested to assess the integrity of the brainstem, particularly in a comatose patient (Table 3-2).

**TABLE 3-2. Brainstem Reflexes and Their Function**

| Reflex | Afferent Nerve | Efferent Nerve | Function |
|---|---|---|---|
| Pupillary reflex | II | III | Shine light—constriction of pupil |
| Corneal reflex | V | VII | Blink to tactile stimuli of cornea |
| Oculocephalic reflex; Oculovestibular reflex | VIII | III, VI | Maintenance of eyes midline with turning of head to left and right<br>May also use caloric testing by flushing cold water into each ear and see deviation of eyes ipsilaterally |
| Response to pain | V | VII | Grimace to painful stimuli (eg intranasal stimuli) |
| Gag reflex | IX | X | Pharyngeal contraction after stimulating the pharynx with a tongue depressor |
| Cough reflex | IX | X | Presence of cough after stimulation of the carina by a bronchial catheter |

## MENINGES

From exterior to interior, the brain sits and is protected within the dura mater, arachnoid layer, and pia mater.

The **falx cerebri** separates the hemispheres and the tentorium cerebelli separates the posterior fossa (cerebellum) from the anterior fossa.

- **Dura mater:** Thickest; composed of irregular, dense connective tissue that adheres to the skull.
  - Epidural hemorrhage follows suture lines, whereas subdural brain bleeds do not.
- **Arachnoid mater:** Fine, weblike avascular membrane directly below the dura.
- **Pia mater:** Delicate innermost layer of the meninges, adherent to brain tissue.

## VENTRICULAR SYSTEM

- CSF produced in choroid plexus in the lateral ventricles → foramen of Monro → third ventricle → sylvian aqueduct → fourth ventricle → foramina of Lushka and Magendie → into subarachnoid space → up to arachnoid granulations to be reabsorbed into venous blood flow (Fig. 3-3).

Performed at L2-L3 or below as the cord ends at L1-L2. Usually performed at L3-L4.

- Normal intracranial pressure (ICP) is 6 to 25 cm $H_2O$.
- Increased ICP can be seen in infection, pseudotumor cerebri/IIH. (Normal pressure is seen in NPH.)

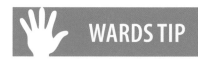

**WARDS TIP**

An important aspect of performing an LP is positioning of the patient.

**KEY FACT**

Hydrocephalus can be communicating (no obstruction and possibly due to impaired resorption by arachnoid granules) or noncommunicating (an obstruction blocking flow at any point).

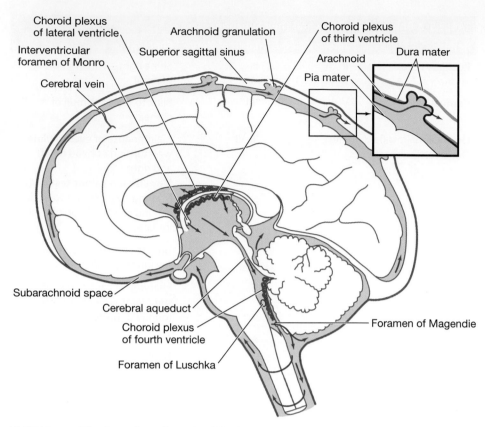

**FIGURE 3-3. The flow of cerebrospinal fluid.** Reproduced with permission from Aminoff MJ, Greenberg, DA, Simaon RP. *Clinical Neurology, 10th ed.* New York: McGraw Hill, 2017.

## Cranial Nerves

The 12 cranial nerves:

- Are specialized and provide motor and sensory functions to the head and neck.
- Are considered part of the peripheral nervous system.
- Can be sensory, motor, or both (Table 3-3).

### TABLE 3-3. Cranial Nerves and Their Associated Functions

#### Cranial Nerves

| Nerve | CN | Function | Type | Mnemonic |
|-------|----|----------|------|----------|
| Olfactory | I | Smell (only CN without thalamic relay to cortex) | **S**ensory | **S**ome |
| Optic | II | Sight | **S**ensory | **S**ay |
| Oculomotor | III | Eye movement (SR, IR, MR, IO), pupillary constriction (sphincter pupillae: Edinger-Westphal nucleus, muscarinic receptors), accommodation, eyelid opening (levator palpebrae) | **M**otor | **M**arry |
| Trochlear | IV | Eye movement (SO) | **M**otor | **M**oney |
| Trigeminal | V | Mastication, facial sensation (ophthalmic, maxillary, mandibular divisions), somatosensation from anterior two-thirds of tongue | **B**oth | **B**ut |

(continued)

**TABLE 3-3. (Continued)**

**Cranial Nerves**

| Nerve | CN | Function | Type | Mnemonic |
|---|---|---|---|---|
| Abducens | VI | Eye movement (LR) | **M**otor | **M**y |
| Facial | VII | Facial movement, taste from anterior two-thirds of tongue, lacrimation, salivation (submandibular and sublingual glands), eyelid closing (orbicularis oculi), auditory volume modulation (stapedius) | **B**oth | **B**rother |
| Vestibulocochlear | VIII | Hearing, balance | **S**ensory | **S**ays |
| Glossopharyngeal | IX | Taste and sensation from posterior one-third of tongue, swallowing, salivation (parotid gland), monitoring carotid body and sinus chemo- and baroreceptors, and elevation of pharynx/larynx (stylopharyngeus) | **B**oth | **B**ig |
| Vagus | X | Taste from supraglottic region, swallowing, soft palate elevation, midline uvula, talking, cough reflex, parasympathetics to thoracoabdominal viscera, monitoring aortic arch chemo- and baroreceptors | **B**oth | **B**rain |
| Accessory | XI | Head turning, shoulder shrugging (SCM, trapezius) | **M**otor | **M**atter |
| Hypoglossal | XII | Tongue movement | **M**otor | **M**ost |

Reproduced with permission from T Le, V Bhushan et.al., *First Aid for the USMLE Step 1, 27th ed.* McGraw Hill, 2017.

## Deep Structures

Deep structures comprise thalamus (Table 3-4), hypothalamus (Table 3-5), and pituitary gland (Table 3-6).

**Thalamus**—Serves as the main relay for all ascending sensory information except olfaction.

**TABLE 3-4. Thalamic Nuclei and Their Functions**

| Nucleus | Input | Senses | Destination | Mnemonic |
|---|---|---|---|---|
| **V**entral **P**ostero-**L**ateral nucleus | Spinothalamic and dorsal columns/medial lemniscus | **V**ibration, **P**ain, **P**ressure, **P**roprioception, **L**ight touch, temperature | 1° somatosensory cortex | |
| Ventral postero-**M**edial nucleus | Trigeminal and gustatory pathway | **Face** sensation, taste | 1° somatosensory cortex | Makeup goes on the **face** |
| **L**ateral geniculate nucleus | CN II | Vision | Calcarine sulcus | **L**ateral = **L**ight |
| **M**edial **G**eniculate nucleus | Superior olive and inferior colliculus of tectum | Hearing | Auditory cortex of temporal lobe | **M**edial = **M**usic |
| Ventral lateral nucleus | Basal ganglia, cerebellum | Motor | Motor cortex | |

Reproduced with permission from T Le, V Bhushan et.al., *First Aid for the USMLE Step 1, 27th ed.* McGraw Hill, 2017.

**Hypothalamus**—Coordinates both the autonomic nervous system and the activity of the pituitary, controlling body temperature, thirst, hunger, and other homeostatic systems, and involved in sleep and emotional activity.

**Pituitary Gland**—The "master gland" releases numerous hormones.

## TABLE 3-5. Hypothalamic Nuclei and Their Functions

| | | |
|---|---|---|
| Hypothalamus | Maintains homeostasis by regulating **T**hirst and water balance, controlling **A**denohypophysis (anterior pituitary) and **N**eurohypophysis (posterior pituitary) release of hormones produced in the hypothalamus, and regulating **H**unger, **A**utonomic nervous system, **T**emperature, and **S**exual urges (**TAN HATS**).<br><br>Inputs (areas not protected by blood-brain barrier): OVLT (senses change in osmolarity), area postrema (found in medulla, responds to emetics). | |
| Lateral area | Hunger. Destruction → anorexia. Stimulated by ghrelin, inhibited by leptin. | If you damage **lateral** area, you shrink **lateral**ly. |
| Ventromedial area | Satiety. Destruction (eg, craniopharyngioma) → hyperphagia. Stimulated by leptin. | If you damage your **ventromedial** area, you grow **ventral**ly and **medial**ly. |
| Anterior hypothalamus | Cooling, parasympathetic. | **Anterior** nucleus = cool off (**cooling**, p**A**rasympathetic). **A/C**= **anterior cooling**. |
| Posterior hypothalamus | Heating, sympathetic. | Posterior nucleus = get fired up (heating, sympathetic). If you injure your **p**osterior hypothalamus, you become a **p**oikilotherm (cold-blooded, like a snake). |
| Suprachiasmatic nucleus | Circadian rhythm. | You need **sleep** to be **charismatic** (chiasmatic). |
| Supraoptic and paraventricular nuclei | Synthesize ADH and oxytocin. | ADH and oxytocin are carried by neurophysins down axons to posterior pituitary, where these hormones are stored and released. |

Reproduced with permission from T Le, V Bhushan et.al., *First Aid for the USMLE Step 1, 27th ed.* McGraw Hill, 2017.

## TABLE 3-6. Anterior and Posterior Divisions of the Pituitary

### Pituitary Gland

| | | |
|---|---|---|
| Anterior pituitary (adenohypophysis) | Secretes FSH, LH, ACTH, TSH, prolactin, GH. Melanotropin (MSH) secreted from intermediate lobe of pituitary. Derived from oral ectoderm (Rathke pouch):<br>• A-subunit—hormone subunit common to TSH, LH, FSH, and hCG.<br>• B-subunit—determines hormone specificity. | ACTH and MSH are derivatives of proopiomelanocortin (POMC). **FLAT PiG**: **F**SH, **L**H, **A**CTH, **T**SH, **P**RL, **G**H.<br>**B-FLAT**: **B**asophils—**F**SH, **L**H, **A**CTH, **T**SH.<br>Acidophils: GH, PRL. |
| Posterior pituitary (neurohypophysis) | Stores and releases vasopressin (antidiuretic hormone, or ADH) and oxytocin, both made in the hypothalamus (supraoptic and paraventricular nuclei) and transported to posterior pituitary via neurophysins (carrier proteins). Derived from neuroectoderm. | |

Reproduced with permission from T Le, V Bhushan et.al., *First Aid for the USMLE Step 1, 27th ed.* McGraw Hill, 2017.

## KEY FACT

Pituitary Adenoma—Present with compressive symptoms late (headaches, visual loss) if they are nonsecretory. Hemorrhage or infarct of the tumor may produce pituitary apoplexy (abrupt headache, visual loss, diplopia, drowsiness, coma). Most common type of pituitary adenoma is prolactinoma.

## Spinal Cord

- Divided into cervical, thoracic, lumbar, and sacral (Fig. 3-4).
- Cord itself terminates in L1-L2 level of lumbar spine.

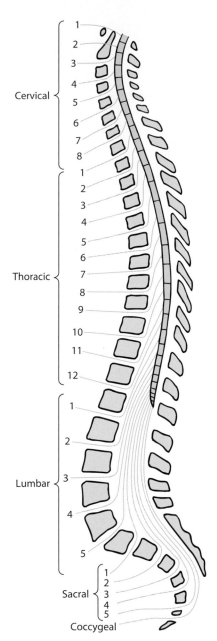

**FIGURE 3-4. Structure of the spinal cord.** Reproduced, with permission, from Waxman SG. *Clinical Neuroanatomy, 25th ed.* New York: McGraw-Hill, 2003.

- Nerves entering and exiting the spinal cord are considered part of the peripheral nervous system.
- This lowest part of the spinal cord is called the conus medullaris (Table 3-7).
- On cross-section, the spinal cord is organized somatotopically (Fig. 3-5).

| TABLE 3-7. Cauda Equina and Conus Medullaris Syndromes | | | | | |
|---|---|---|---|---|---|
| | Level of Lesion | Weakness | Sensory Deficit | Reflexes | Bowel/Bladder Involvement |
| **Cauda equina** Onset: Gradual asymmetric | L4, L5, or S1 | Asymmetric | Asymmetric saddle anesthesia in all modalities | Ankle jerk absent Knee jerk absent | Retention, develops later Decreased rectal tone |
| **Conus medullaris** Onset: Sudden bilateral | L1, L2 | Symmetric | Symmetric saddle anesthesia in small fiber | Ankle jerk absent Knee jerk preserved | Incontinence Develops early |

Reproduced with permission from Rafii M, Thomas C. *First Aid for the Neurology Boards, 2nd ed.* New York: McGraw Hill, 2015.

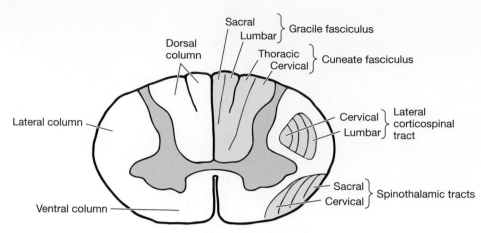

**FIGURE 3-5. Somatotopic organization of the spinal cord.** Reproduced with permission from Waxman SG. *Clinical Neuroanatomy, 25th ed.* New York: McGraw-Hill, 2003.

■ The levels of the spinal cord stay consistent with levels of vertebral bodies until the Lumbar spine where the cord levels are much shorter than the large lumbar vertebral bodies.

■ While the spinal cord and vertebral bodies are not completely aligned vertically, the spinal nerves exit from their respective levels in the cord and course down the spinal canal to exit the canal beneath their respective vertebral bodies.

■ These nerves which traverse the spinal canal outside the cord form a "tail" and are called the *cauda equina (horse tail).*

The peripheral white matter houses axons which travel vertically and synapse with motor neurons which are in the gray matter.

■ Axial muscles are innervated by somatic motor neurons which travel in the medial motor columns.

■ Upper and lower extremities are innervated by somatic motor neurons which travel in the lateral motor columns.

■ Somatic and visceral afferent (sensory) fibers enter the dorsal horn with their cell bodies in the dorsal root ganglion (DRG) which lies outside the spinal cord.

■ Autonomic neurons originate in the spinal cord.

• Cell bodies of the sympathetic preganglionic neurons are located in C8 through L1. Parasympathetic preganglionic cell bodies in S2 through S4. These bodies lie in the intermediolateral and intermediomedial columns.

## SPINAL CORD PATHWAYS

■ **Ascending posterior column-medial lemniscal (PC/ML) pathway (Fig. 3-6):**

• Transmits vibration, proprioception, fine touch from periphery to brain. Enters spinal cord ipsilaterally → ascends in posterior column → crosses in caudal medulla into medial lemniscus → ventral posterior lateral nucleus of thalamus → primary somatosensory cortex.

Two important conditions that can affect the dorsal columns:

■ **Tabes dorsalis:**

• Neurologic sequelae associated with **tertiary syphilis**

• Degeneration of dorsal columns

• Loss of proprioception, light touch, and vibratory sensation

---

## WARDS TIP

Cauda Equina syndrome often presents with gradual bladder/bowels incontinence, altered sensation between the legs or over the buttocks, the inner thighs, the back of the legs, the feet or the heels. Pain, numbness, or weakness in one or both legs.

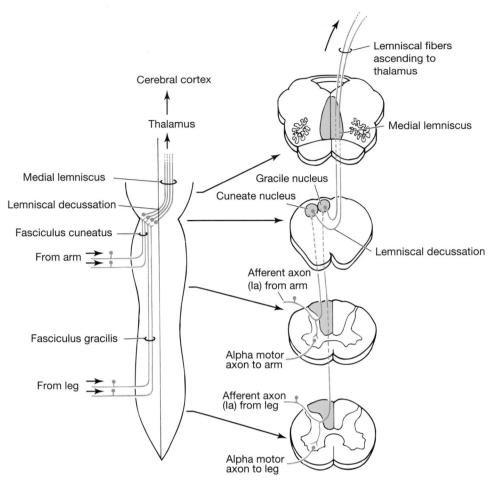

**FIGURE 3-6. Dorsal column/medial lemniscus pathway.** Reproduced, with permission, from Waxman SG. *Clinical Neuroanatomy, 25th ed.* New York: McGraw-Hill, 2003.

- **Subacute combined degeneration:**
  - **B12 deficiency** (pernicious anemia, nitrous oxide use). B12 deficiency begins with damage to dorsal columns and progresses to damage of corticospinal tract leading to weakness.

### Ascending anterolateral (also called spinothalamic) pathway (Fig. 3-7):

- Transmits pain, temperature, crude touch.
- Enters ipsilaterally, will rise as far as two levels ipsilaterally before decussating → ascending in anterolateral portion of spinal cord → ventral posterior lateral nucleus of thalamus → primary sensory cortex.
- Lesions to the spinal cord will damage pain/temperature on contralateral body starting two levels below level of lesion.

### Brown-Sequard syndrome:

- Complete transverse hemisection of spinal cord
- Trauma (eg, stab wounds to neck), tumors, inflammation/infection, hematoma, degenerative disk disease
- Contralateral loss of pain, temperature, crude touch starting TWO levels below lesion
- Ipsilateral loss of proprioception, light touch, and vibration sense below level of lesion

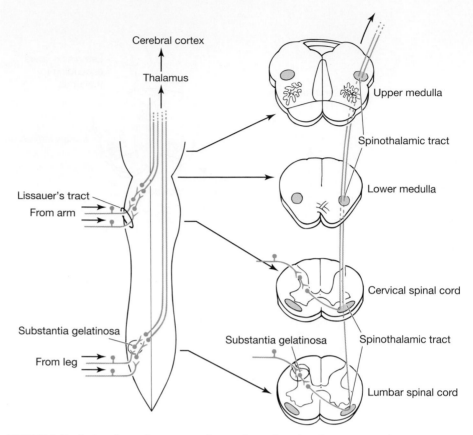

**FIGURE 3-7. Anterolateral system pathway.** Reproduced, with permission, from Waxman SG. *Clinical Neuroanatomy, 25th ed.* New York: McGraw-Hill, 2003.

- Motor paralysis with UMN signs below level of lesion and LMN injury at level of lesion
- Some ipsilateral sensory loss at level of lesion

**Descending tracts:**

- **Corticospinal tract:** Primary motor cortex → internal capsule → cerebral peduncles of midbrain → base of pons → medullary pyramids with decussation at caudal medulla → lateral corticospinal tract → motor neurons in anterior horn → muscle.
- Corticospinal lesions result in a classic presentation (Fig. 3-8).
  - There is more weakness in extensors in UE and flexors in LE.
  - Patient's arm is flexed and leg is extended.
- **Rubrospinal** tract originates from red nucleus in midbrain.
  - An extrapyramidal tract which is involved in control of balance.
  - Lesions to descending motor tracts above red nucleus allow this pathway to be un-antagonized, resulting in **decorticate** posturing: bent arms, clenched fists, and legs held out straight = flexor posturing.
  - In contrast, decerebrate posturing the arms and legs being held straight out, the toes being pointed downward, and the head and neck being arched backward in which the lesion is below the red nucleus and patients exhibit extensor posturing.
- **Reticulospinal** tract sends motor information from reticular formation in brainstem.
- **Tectospinal** tract coordinates head and eye movements.
- **Vestibulospinal** tract sends balance information from vestibular system to the extremities.

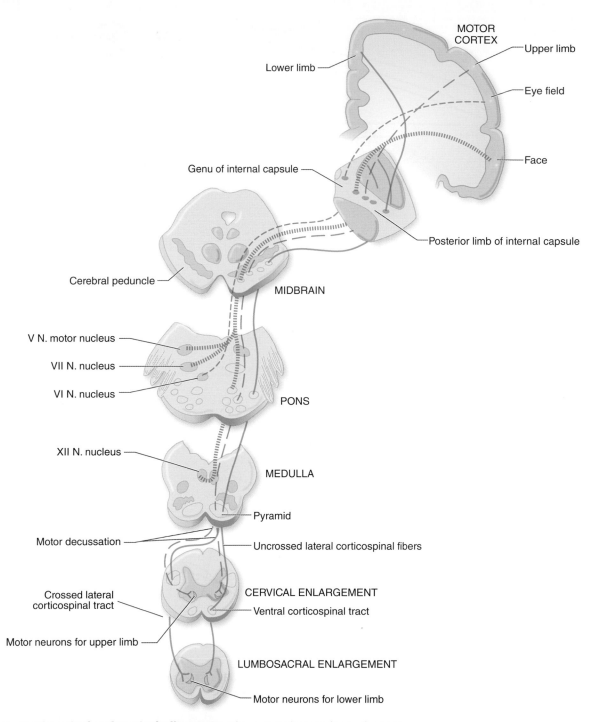

FIGURE 3-8. **Corticospinal and corticobulbar tracts.** The various lines indicate the trajectories of these pathways, from their origin in particular parts of the cerebral cortex to their nuclei of termination. Reproduced with permission from Ropper AH, Samuels MA, et al., *Adams and Victor's Principles of Neurology, 11th ed.* New York: McGraw Hill, 2019.

## Autonomic Nervous System (Fig. 3-9)

- Sympathetic nervous system primary neurons derived from hypothalamus travels down to spinal cord as the hypothalamospinal tract and exits in thoracolumbar region (T1-L2) with ganglia outside the spinal cord.

- Parasympathetic nervous system exits through brainstem and sacral cord.

- Descending fibers from the pontine micturition center synapse on preganglionic neurons in lumbar spine.

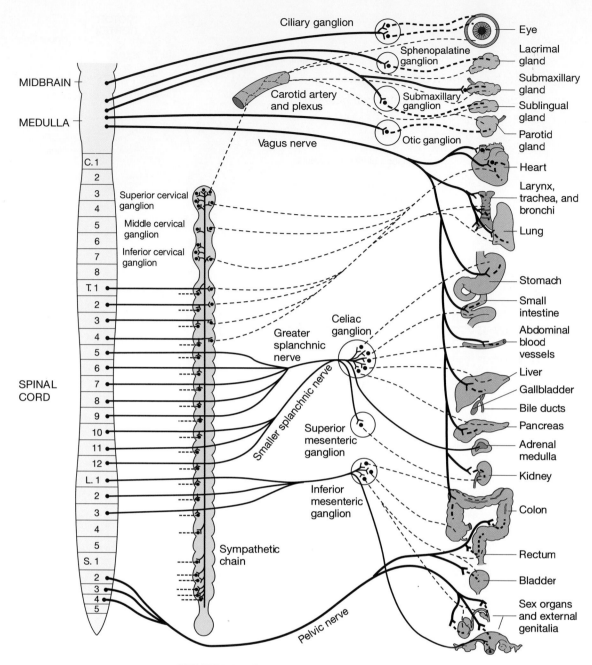

**FIGURE 3-9. The autonomic nervous system and its sympathetic and parasympathetic divisions.** Reproduced with permission from WF Ganong. *Review of Medical Physiology, 22nd ed.* New York. McGraw-Hill, 2005.

**KEY FACT**

Control of the urinary bladder is both sympathetic and parasympathetic.

- Injury anywhere in this pathway leads to uncontrolled parasympathetic activity and overactive bladder.
- Injury to sacral cord/parasympathetic pathway results in urinary retention and can manifest as retention as well as incontinence d/t overflow (with incomplete emptying).
- Damage to cervical spinal cord can lead to long-term reliance on ventilator.
  - Damage to phrenic nerve *(C3, C4, C5 keeps the diaphragm alive).*

Other cord syndromes:
- **Central cord syndrome:**
  - Distal > proximal weakness in upper limbs (especially hands)

- Upper > lower limbs
- Bladder dysfunction and priapism
- **Capelike** sensory loss to pain and temperature in upper trunk and arms at level of lesion (often seen in **Syringomyelia**)
- Patchy loss of pain, temperature, light touch below lesion
- Preservation of sacral and lower limb sensation because these spinothalamic tracts run laterally

■ **Anterior cord syndrome:**
  - Motor weakness
  - Loss of pain and temperature below lesion
  - Proprioception and vibration preserved

■ **Posterior cord syndrome:**
  - Sensory ataxia
  - Proprioceptive deficits
  - Vibration deficits

### Stretch reflex:

■ The **golgi apparatus** in the tendon of the targeted muscle sends a stretch signal via the afferent fiber to the dorsal column → direct synapse onto motor neuron of struck muscle and indirect connection via inhibitory interneuron to antagonist muscle.

### Symptoms of spinal cord lesion:

■ Bilateral > unilateral motor and/or sensory symptoms

■ Bladder, bowel, sexual dysfunction

■ Retention or hyperactive

■ Stiffness in legs

■ Neck or back pain with neurological deficits (especially in presence of trauma)

### Neurogenic claudication:

■ Painful cramping or weakness in legs with walking and improves with rest.

### Syringomyelia:

■ Expansion of central canal by fluid-filled cyst. Usually cervical, and often after trauma to neck.

■ Can be associated with Chiari malformation, tumors, trauma, inflammation.

■ Bilateral loss of spinothalamic fibers at level of lesion ("cape-like" distribution).

■ Lower motor neuron weakness in hands and upper motor neuron weakness in legs (Fig. 3-10).

### Vascular supply of the spinal cord:

■ The blood supply to the spinal cord is important in understanding how a patient may present with an interruption in blood supply.

■ Anterior spinal artery and posterior spinal arteries branch from the vertebral arteries branch at the cervical-cranial junction.

## KEY FACT

Syringomyelia is when a fluid-filled cavity or cyst (syrinx) forms within the spinal cord and compresses spinal pathways.

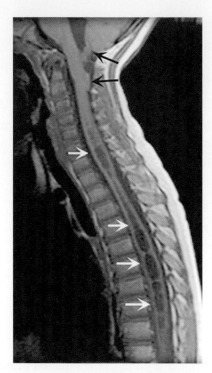

**FIGURE 3-10. Syringomyelia (a syrinx) is seen on sagittal cervical MRI.** Sagittal T1-weighted image through the cervical and upper thoracic spine demonstrates descent of the cerebellar tonsils below the level of the foramen magnum (*black arrows*). Within the substance of the cervical and thoracic spinal cord, a cerebrospinal fluid collection dilates the central canal (*white arrows*). Reprinted, with permission, from Loscalzo J, Fauci A, Kasper D, Hauser S, Longo D, Jameson J, eds. *Harrison's Principles of Internal Medicine, 21st ed.* New York, NY: McGraw Hill; 2022: Figure 442-7.

KEY FACT

Artery of Adamkiewicz (aka the great anterior radiculomedullary artery) anastomotically supplies the anterior spinal artery between T9 and T12. Supplies the cord from T9 to conus medullaris.

- Also receive supply from the cervical arteries from the thyrocervical trunk.
- Thyrocervical trunk also gives rise to radiculomedullary arteries which supply cervical spinal cord; radiculomedullary arteries which supply the thoracolumbar spinal cord come from the aorta.
- The anterior spinal artery supplies anterior two-thirds of the spinal cord including the ventral horns, corticospinal tract, anterolateral spinal tracts, autonomic cell bodies.
- Posterior spinal arteries supply posterior one-third which is the dorsal columns (vibration, proprioception).
- Venous drainage: dorsal and ventral spinal veins → internal and external venous plexi which are next to dural sac and vertebral bodies → dural venous sinuses.

## Peripheral Nervous System

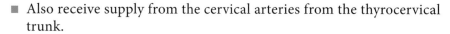

- Consists of motor, sensory, and autonomic nerves.
  - Oligodendrocytes are in the CNS, while Schwann cells are in peripheral nervous system (PNS). Both serve to myelinate neurons.
  - The sensory endings in the skin each detect a certain kind of sensation (see Table 3-8) and transmit these sensations via the ascending sensory tracts (Figs. 3-11 and 3-12).

## TABLE 3-8. Frequently Tested Muscle Groups and Their Anatomical Correlations

| Muscle | Innervation | Function |
|---|---|---|
| Deltoid | **C5**, axillary nerve | Shoulder abduction |
| Biceps | C5-**C6**, musculocutaneous nerve | Elbow flexion |
| Triceps | **C7**-C8, radial nerve | Elbow extension |
| Extensor carpi radialis | **C5-C6**, radial nerve | Wrist extension |
| Abductor pollicis brevis | **C8-T1,** median nerve | Palmar adduction of thumb |
| Iliopsoas | **L3**, femoral nerve | Hip flexion |
| Quadriceps | L2-L4, femoral nerve | Knee extension |
| Hamstrings | L4-L5, mainly tibial nerve | Knee flexion |
| Gastrocnemius/soleus | **S1**-S2, tibial nerve | Ankle plantarflexion |
| Tibialis anterior | **L5**, deep peroneal nerve | Ankle dorsiflexion |

| Sensory System | Modality | Stimulus | Receptor Class | Receptor Cell Type |
|---|---|---|---|---|
| Somatosensory | Touch | Tap, flutter 5–40 Hz | Cutaneous mechanoreceptor | Meissner corpuscle |
| Somatosensory | Touch | Motion | Cutaneous mechanoreceptor | Hair follicle receptor |
| Somatosensory | Touch | Vibration 60–500 Hz; deep pressure | Cutaneous mechanoreceptor | Pacinian corpuscle |
| Somatosensory | Touch | Touch, sustained pressure | Cutaneous mechanoreceptor | Merkel cell |
| Somatosensory | Touch | Skin stretch, vibration | Cutaneous mechanoreceptor | Ruffini corpuscle |
| Somatosensory | Proprioception | Stretch | Mechanoreceptor | Muscle spindle |
| Somatosensory | Proprioception | Tension | Mechanoreceptor | Golgi tendon organ |
| Somatosensory | Temperature | Thermal | Thermoreceptor | Cold and warm receptors |
| Somatosensory | Pain | Chemical, thermal, and mechanical | Chemoreceptor, thermoreceptor, and mechanoreceptor | Polymodal receptors or chemical, thermal, and mechanical nociceptors |
| Somatosensory | Itch | Chemical | Chemoreceptor | Chemical nociceptor |
| Visual | Vision | Light | Photoreceptor | Rods, cones |
| Auditory | Hearing | Sound | Mechanoreceptor | Hair cells (cochlea) |
| Vestibular | Balance | Angular acceleration | Mechanoreceptor | Hair cells (semicircular canals) |
| Vestibular | Balance | Linear acceleration, gravity | Mechanoreceptor | Hair cells (otolith organs) |
| Olfactory | Smell | Chemical | Chemoreceptor | Olfactory sensory neuron |
| Gustatory | Taste | Chemical | Chemoreceptor | Taste buds |

**FIGURE 3-11. Cutaneous receptors and the sensation that they convey.** Reproduced with permission from Somatosensory neurotransmission: Touch, pain, & temperature. In: Barrett KE, Barman SM, Brooks HL, Yuan JJ, eds. *Ganong's Review of Medical Physiology, 26th ed.* New York, NY: McGraw Hill; 2019.

| | Motor Neuron Disease | Neuropathy | Neuromuscular Junction | Myopathy |
|---|---|---|---|---|
| Weakness pattern | Variable | Distal | Diffuse | Proximal |
| Deep tendon reflexes | Increased, normal, or decreased | Decreased or absent | Normal or decreased | Normal or decreased |
| Atrophy | Yes | Yes | No | No |
| Fasciculations | Yes | Sometimes | No | No |
| Sensory symptoms and signs | No | Yes | No | No |

**FIGURE 3-12. Patterns of weakness and associated localization.** Reproduced with permission from Likosky DJ, Josephson S. The neurologic examination. In: McKean SC, Ross JJ, Dressler DD, Scheurer DB, eds. *Principles and Practice of Hospital Medicine, 2nd ed.* New York, NY: McGraw Hill; 2017.

**Case 1:** A 60-year-old man is being examined because of difficulty walking. The clinician notices the presence of fine twitching movements throughout his protruded tongue and wasting of one side. This finding suggests which of the following?

A. Corticobasilar degeneration
B. Denervation of muscles from CN XI
C. Denervation of muscles from CN XII
D. Aberrant reinnervation of muscles from CN XI
E. Aberrant reinnervation of muscles from CN XII

The correct answer is C. The finding is consistent with denervation of CN XII, the hypoglossal nerve. This is a finding concerning for ALS.

**Case 2:** A 30-year-old woman fractures her humerus in a car accident. As the pain from the acute injury subsides, she notices weakness on flexion at the elbow. She also notices paresthesias over the dorsal aspect of the forearm. During the accident, she probably injured which one of the following nerves?

A. Long thoracic nerve
B. Musculocutaneous nerve
C. Radial nerve
D. Suprascapular nerve
E. Ulnar nerve

The correct answer is C. The radial nerve is sensory and innervates the forearm. It would have been the nerve that was injured with a fracture of the humerus.

**Case 3:** A 35-year-old man participated in civil war re-enactments and was injured in his thoracic spine by an accidental bayonet to the back. Initially he had a bilateral spastic paraparesis and urinary urgency, but this has improved. He still has pain and thermal sensation loss on part of his left body and proprioception loss in his right foot. There is still a paralysis of the right lower extremity as well. This patient most likely has which of the following spinal cord conditions?

A. Syringomyelia
B. Brown-Sequard syndrome
C. Tabes Dorsalis
D. Spinal cord ischemia on the left side

The correct answer is B. Hemisection of the spinal cord results in a contralateral loss of pain and thermal sensation due to spinothalamic damage and ipsilateral loss of proprioception due to posterior column damage. He has Brown-Sequard syndrome.

# CHAPTER 4

# CEREBROVASCULAR DISEASE

In this chapter, we will review cerebrovascular anatomy, different types of strokes, and how they present with various signs and symptoms and review their treatment. CT and MRI images are presented to provide examples that may also be seen on the wards and on the shelf exam.

## Arterial Blood Supply to the Brain

The blood supply to the brain, like every other organ, has its roots in the aorta. Branches give rise to the anterior and posterior circulations (Fig. 4-1).

**Anterior circulation** derives blood from the bilateral internal carotid arteries and supplies blood to most of the cerebral hemispheres, including the frontal lobes, parietal lobes, lateral temporal lobes, and anterior part of deep cerebral hemispheres (Figs. 4-2A and 4-2B).

- Begins with the internal carotid arteries (external carotid arteries are extracranial) which migrate up the neck, through the skull and end in the circle of Willis (Fig. 4-3).
  - The circle is completed with smaller (but still very important) communicating arteries. The anterior communicating artery connects left and right anterior cerebral arteries while the posterior communicating artery is important for connecting the anterior circulation to the posterior circulation.
- The anterior cerebral arteries (ACA) supply the most medial, frontal, and rostral parts of the cortex.

### KEY FACT

ACA strokes often result in weakness of the contralateral leg.

### KEY FACT

Four arteries bring blood to the brain, two common carotid arteries and 2 vertebral arteries.

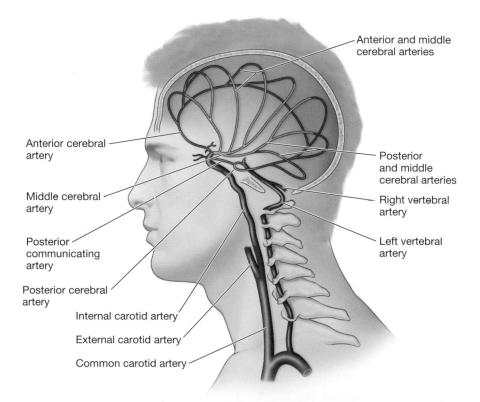

**FIGURE 4-1. Blood supply to the brain—anterior circulation (common carotid arteries) and posterior circulation (vertebral arteries).** Anastomotic channels between the middle and anterior cerebral arteries, and the middle and posterior cerebral arteries are depicted. The left side of the circle of Willis is shown: anterior communicating artery (purple; unlabeled), posterior communicating artery, and posterior cerebral artery. Reproduced with permission from Martin JH, eds. *Neuroanatomy: Text and Atlas, 5th ed.* New York: McGraw Hill; 2021.

**A**

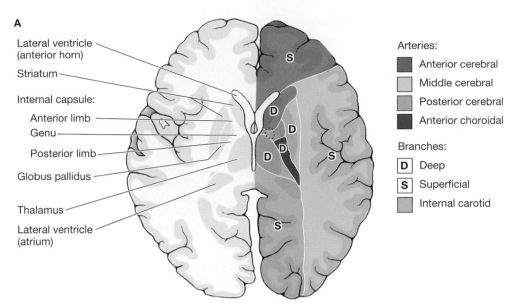

Lateral ventricle (anterior horn)
Striatum
Internal capsule:
Anterior limb
Genu
Posterior limb
Globus pallidus
Thalamus
Lateral ventricle (atrium)

Arteries:
- Anterior cerebral
- Middle cerebral
- Posterior cerebral
- Anterior choroidal

Branches:
- **D** Deep
- **S** Superficial
- Internal carotid

**FIGURE 4-2A. Cortical distribution of cerebral arteries (anterior cerebral arteries, middle cerebral arteries, and posterior cerebral arteries).** Reproduced with permission from Martin JH, eds. *Neuroanatomy: Text and Atlas, 5th ed.* New York: McGraw Hill; 2021.

**B**

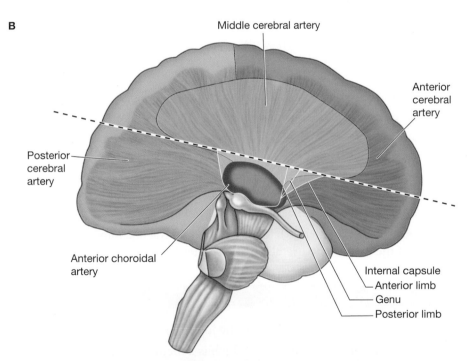

Middle cerebral artery
Anterior cerebral artery
Posterior cerebral artery
Anterior choroidal artery
Internal capsule
Anterior limb
Genu
Posterior limb

**FIGURE 4-2B. Arterial supply of the subcortical white matter and internal capsule.** Different dorsoventral levels of the internal capsule and limbs receive their arterial supply from different cerebral arteries. The dashed line indicates the plane of the horizontal section in Figure 4-2A. The territories supplied by each cerebral artery are shown. Reproduced with permission from Martin JH, eds. *Neuroanatomy: Text and Atlas, 5th ed.* New York: McGraw Hill; 2021.

■ The middle cerebral arteries (MCA) supply the lateral cortices, including the frontal, parietal, and superior temporal lobes.

**Posterior circulation** derives blood from the bilateral vertebral arteries. It supplies the brainstem, cerebellum, occipital lobes, medial temporal lobes, and posterior part of the deep hemisphere, mainly the thalamus.

**KEY FACT**

MCA strokes often are some of the most debilitating as they affect large areas of cortex.

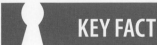

## KEY FACT

Vertebral arteries join to form the Basilar artery.

## KEY FACT

Basilar strokes such as pontine infarct can result in locked-in syndrome (quadriplegia).

## KEY FACT

The posterior communicating artery can have an aneurysm and can cause a CN III palsy which appears first as a dilated pupil and then as it presses on CN III more, a down and out presentation (see below under cranial nerves for how to tell the difference between this and a diabetic third palsy).

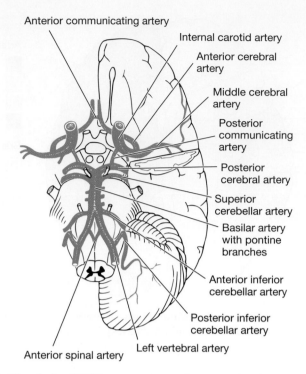

**FIGURE 4-3.** **The circle of Willis, an anastomotic connection between the anterior and posterior circulations, provides collateral flow to affected brain regions in the event of arterial blockage.** Reproduced, with permission, from Ropper AH, Brown RH. *Adams and Victor's Principles of Neurology,* 8th ed. New York: McGraw-Hill, 2003: Figure 12-2.

- Begins with the vertebral arteries which combine to form the basilar artery which then splits into the posterior cerebral arteries (PCAs).
- The posterior inferior cerebellar arteries come off each vertebral artery before forming the basilar artery.
- The basilar artery then gives rise to the major arteries that supply the brainstem and cerebellum: the perforators, anterior-inferior cerebellar artery, and superior cerebellar artery.
- The PCAs supply the inferior temporal lobes and the occipital cortex, as well as parts of the posterior parietal lobe (precuneus).

## Venous Circulation

- Drain blood supply from the brain to the jugular veins.
- At risk for dural venous thrombosis which is a medical emergency (Fig. 4-4).
  - Thrombosis can lead to venous congestion and, in turn, edema-induced infarction (ie, stroke).

## Stroke

It refers to focal neurological deficit(s) secondary to neuron death from interruption of cerebral vessels delivering oxygen and nutrition, whether due to a clot (ischemic) or bleed (hemorrhagic).

### ISCHEMIC STROKE

Occlusion of arterial vessel that leads to cell death and cytotoxic edema.

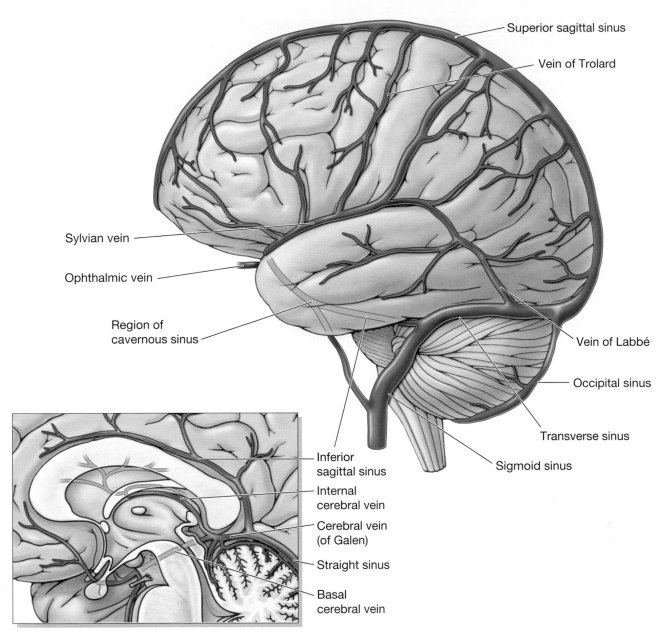

**FIGURE 4-4. Dural venous sinuses.** Lateral view of the brain, showing major superficial veins and the dural sinuses. Inset shows veins on midline. Reproduced with permission from Martin JH, eds. *Neuroanatomy: Text and Atlas, 5th ed.* New York: McGraw Hill; 2021.

## Etiology

- Cardioembolic source
  - Atrial fibrillation
    - Irregularly irregular heart rhythm that is prone to turbulent flow and clot (embolus) formation in the left heart, with subsequent dislodging to cerebral vessels.
  - Patent foramen ovale (PFO)
    - A right-to-left shunt in the heart that allows emboli from venous (right) side of the heart to travel to the arterial (left) circulation.
    - Rule out deep vein thrombosis (DVT) in lower extremities.
    - Look for underlying hypercoagulable or thrombophilic state.

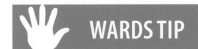

**WARDS TIP**

Anticoagulation is used to prevent embolic strokes due to Afib or PFO.

- Left atrial appendage, left ventricular thrombus in chamber
  - High risk for dislodging to cerebral vessels.
- Valvular disease
  - Bacterial endocarditis could lead to septic emboli. Treating the underlying infection requires long-term antibiotics and possibly surgical repair of the valve.
  - **Libman-Sacks endocarditis** (associated with systemic **lupus** erythematosus) is a form of nonbacterial endocarditis.
- Hypoperfusion: Global drop in blood pressure such as due to cardiac arrest.
- Thromboembolic source
  - Emboli dislodging from focal thrombus on an arterial vessel wall, "artery-to-artery" stroke.
  - Symptomatic or significant focal stenosis in common or internal carotid artery may need endarterectomy or stent.
- Thrombophilic/Hypercoagulable states
  - Inherited thrombophilic states.
  - Protein S, Protein C deficiency, antithrombin deficiency, Factor V Leiden, prothrombin gene mutation.
- Acquired hypercoagulable states
  - Pregnancy, malignancy, immobilization, surgery, trauma, oral contraceptive use, hormonal replacement, antiphospholipid antibody syndrome (lupus anticoagulant, anticardiolipin, anti-$\beta_2$ glycoprotein positive state), polycythemia vera.
- Thrombotic stroke
  - Occlusion of a narrow (stenotic) vessel due to underlying atherosclerosis.
  - Risk factors: Hypertension, cigarette smoking, heart disease, alcohol abuse, diabetes mellitus, vasculitis, fibromuscular dysplasia, Moyamoya disease.
  - Imaging: Focal atherosclerosis and stenosis on CT angiography of vessels, sometimes with concurrent burden of atherosclerosis in other vessels.
- Lacunar infarcts
  - Occlusion of the small, deep penetrating arteries of the brain. Also, possibly secondary to embolic or thrombotic etiology.
  - Imaging: Hypodensity in the deep areas of the brain on CT.
- Systemic hypoperfusion
  - Due to global hypoperfusion, most often secondary to cardiac arrest or shock.
  - Imaging: Border zone (watershed) infarcts.
  - Watershed infarcts (Fig. 4-5)
    - Ischemic stroke involving the watershed region between two vascular territories due to focal or generalized reduction in perfusion pressure.
    - Most commonly occurs between the MCA and ACA territories → bilateral infarcts along the medial cortical and subcortical regions → bilateral proximal arm/leg and trunk weakness.
    - Occurs with systemic hypotension or focal arterial stenosis/occlusion.
- Other etiologies of strokes

**KEY FACT**

Some embolic strokes are *cryptogenic or of unknown source,* meaning there was no clear etiology in the workup.

**KEY FACT**

"Symptomatic" internal carotid stenosis: **Transient Ischemic Attack** (TIA) or stroke due to ICA stenosis of 50% to 99% should be treated with endarterectomy.

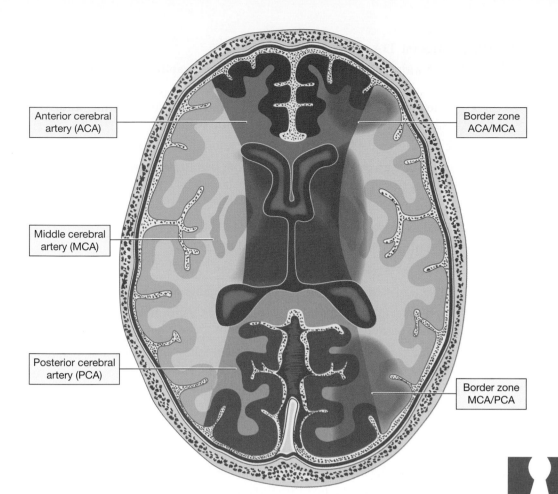

**FIGURE 4-5. Border zone or "watershed" infarcts.** The watershed zones are vulnerable because they are situated furthest away from the major arteries that supply the brain.

- Fibromuscular dysplasia
  - Internal carotid artery stenosis that could lead to aneurysm or dissection.
  - Concurrent with renal artery stenosis.
  - Hyperplasia seen as beading pattern similar to vasculitis.
  - Moyamoya disease.

## PRIMARY CENTRAL NERVOUS SYSTEM (CNS) VASCULITIS

- **Etiology**: Autoimmune, inflammatory disease of medium- and small-caliber cerebral arteries in the absence of other systemic vasculitic manifestations.
  **Symptoms:** Subacute presentation of headache and progressive/stepwise neurological deficits.
- Onset usually in 40s and 50s.
- May have nonspecific markers of inflammation such as elevated ESR.
- MRI shows nonspecific white matter disease and is rarely normal.
- Angiography may show "beading" of blood vessels similar to vasospasm.
- Brain and meningeal biopsy is gold standard but still only ~75% sensitive.

## TRANSIENT ISCHEMIC ATTACK (TIA)

- Stroke symptoms that resolve within 24 hours
- ABCD$^2$ score for risk stratification of subsequent stroke after TIA
- Same workup as for stroke

**Diagnostics for TIA or stroke:**

■ CT head without contrast ± perfusion, CT angiography head and neck with contrast:

- Acute infarct is hypodense (dark) compared to the surrounding brain tissue but not as dark as cerebrospinal fluid (CSF).

- Chronic infarcts (encephalomalacia or gliosis) may appear as dark as CSF.

- Perfusion scan can delineate infarct from penumbra (tissue with low perfusion at risk of stroke but still salvageable).

■ MRI brain without contrast (Fig. 4-6):

- Stroke sequence, diffusion restriction:

  - **W**hite on **D**iffusion **W**eighted **I**maging (DWI).

  - **D**ark on **A**pparent **D**iffusion **C**oefficient (ADC).

■ Transthoracic echocardiogram (TTE) with bubble study and contrast:

- Can detect right to left cardiac shunt like PFO, thrombus, valvular disease, and contractility.

- If highly concerning for endocarditis, then follow up with a transesophageal echocardiogram (TEE) even if TTE is negative.

- Heart failure or low left ventricular ejection fraction could also increase chance of ischemic stroke.

■ Electrocardiogram (EKG):

- Monitor for myocardial infarction which leads to poor heart contraction and thus compromised cerebral perfusion.

- Monitor for abnormal heart rhythms such as atrial fibrillation or flutter that put the patient at high risk for cardioembolic phenomenon.

■ Labs for stroke risk factors:

- Blood glucose (BG), Hgb A1c, thyroid stimulating hormone (TSH), lipid panel.

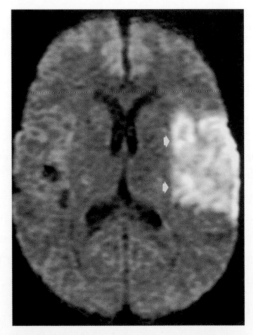

**FIGURE 4-6. Acute left middle cerebral artery infarct on MRI of a 65-year-old hypertensive man.** The MRI demonstrates increased signal intensity (arrows). Abnormalities in MRI occur before those seen on CT during ischemic strokes. Reproduced, with permission, from Chen MYM, Pope TL, Ott DJ. *Basic Radiology.* New York, NY: McGraw-Hill Education; 2004.

- The caliber of vessels matter:
  - Small vessel (lacunar) stroke: Perforators in basal ganglia from the middle cerebral arteries and pons from the basilar artery.
  - Large vessel occlusion: Occlusion in a major cerebral artery such as proximal MCA, ACA, basilar, or PCA.

### Management of acute ischemic stroke:

- Intravenous (IV) thrombolysis:
  - IV tissue plasminogen activator (tPA) such as alteplase or tenecteplase if within 4.5-hour window of last known well time and without contraindications.
  - Post-IV thrombolysis monitoring in the ICU for serial vitals, neurological checks, and repeat imaging in 24 hours.
- Blood pressure management:
  - Without thrombolysis: permissive hypertension to allow systolic blood pressure (SBP) <220 mm Hg, diastolic blood pressure (DBP) <110 mm Hg for first 24 hours for optimal cerebral perfusion.
  - With thrombolysis: SBP <180 mm Hg, DBP <105 mm Hg.
- Endovascular intervention:
  - Could be considered for large-vessel occlusions that are amenable and timely.
  - Mechanical thrombectomy for large-vessel occlusion in 24-hour window (ideally 6 hours).
  - Symptomatic stenosis in a large vessel such as internal carotid artery may need additional interventions such as endarterectomy, stenting, or bypass more urgently.
- Secondary prevention:
  - Antithrombotic agents such as aspirin, clopidogrel, etc., or combination/dual antiplatelet therapy.
  - Statin.
  - Anticoagulation when indicated:
    - Atrial fibrillation/flutter:
      - Valvular afib: Concurrent moderate-to-severe mitral or aortic disease or mechanical valve require coumadin.
      - Nonvalvular afib: Direct oral anticoagulation.
    - PFO closure for young patients with recurrent strokes.
    - Hypercoagulable state.

## HEMORRHAGIC STROKE

- Etiologies: Hypertension, trauma.
- Clinical characteristics: Bleeding of arterial or venous cerebral vessel.
- Diagnostics:
  - CT head without contrast and CT angiography head with contrast.
    - Acute blood is hyperdense (bright).
    - Obtain stability scan in 6 hours to monitor hematoma expansion.

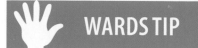

**WARDS TIP**

**Stroke code checklist**
- Last seen normal/time of symptom onset
- National Institutes of Health Stroke Scale score (NIHSS)
- Blood glucose
- Systolic blood pressure (SBP)
- Weight
- CT scan of head
- Candidacy for IV thrombolysis or endovascular intervention

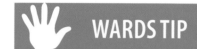

**WARDS TIP**

**Check list for tPA (IV thrombolysis) (abridged)**
- Must know BP and BG before considering IV thrombolysis
- SBP <185 mm Hg; DBP <110 mm Hg
- BG >50
- And
- No major surgery within 14 days
- No major active bleed
- No stroke within 3 months
- INR <1.7
- Platelet >100k

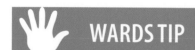

**WARDS TIP**

Standard workup of stroke typically includes MRI, vessel imaging with CT, MR, or carotid ultrasound, and echocardiogram.

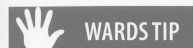

**WARDS TIP**

What is bright on CT? The four Bs: Bullets, Bones, Blood, Bontrast (contrast).

- Management:
  - Blood pressure control and monitoring for clinical signs of elevated intracranial pressure (ICP) in the Intensive Care Unit ± intracranial pressure monitor.
  - Serial neurological checks.
  - Surgical intervention when indicated.

Other causes of intracerebral hemorrhage:

**Cerebral amyloid angiopathy:** Deposition of beta-amyloid in the media and adventitia of small- and medium-sized arteries of the cerebral cortex and meninges.

Risk factors: Advanced age (typically 80s), Alzheimer dementia, Down syndrome (earlier onset).

Typical presentation: New ICH in patient with dementia; cortical or lobar ICH in the absence of significant hypertension; silent cortical microbleeds seen best on gradient echo or susceptibility-weighted MRI sequences.

**Arteriovenous malformation (AVM):** Tangle of abnormal, tortuous arteriovenous fistulas that lack an intervening capillary bed and are separated by a nidus of brain tissue; most commonly supratentorial (extending from subcortical region to the ventricle in a wedge shape) but can occur anywhere; patients present with headache, seizures, or hemorrhage; 2% annual hemorrhage rate, 10% to 20% recurrence rate in first year after hemorrhage; best seen on MRI.

**Cavernous hemangioma:** Cluster of thin-walled veins without significant arterial feeders or intervening brain tissue; infratentorial in 50%, multiple in 10%, and familial (autosomal dominant) in 5%; hemorrhage rate 1% to 2%/year; best seen on MRI.

**Underlying tumor:** Most common metastatic tumors that bleed are breast, lung, thyroid, renal cell, melanoma, and choriocarcinoma.

**Subarachnoid hemorrhage (SAH) (Fig. 4-7):**
- Etiologies: Trauma, rupture of aneurysm, AVM.
- Clinical characteristics: Sudden onset, worst in lifetime thunderclap headaches; seizures.
- Imaging characteristics (CT): Star of David/Starfish sign with hyperdensity along the cortex and in between the sulci; hydrocephalus.
- CSF will show elevated RBCs and xanthochromia (yellowish appearance of CSF that occurs several hours after bleeding into the subarachnoid space).

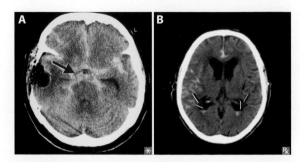

**FIGURE 4-7. CT demonstrating SAH (A) with ventricular extension (B).**

■ Management:
- Blood pressure control (SBP <140 mm Hg).
- Nimodipine to prevent vasospasm.
- External ventricular drain (EVD) if resulting in intraventricular extension and concerning for elevated ICP from hydrocephalus.
- Clipping or coiling of the underlying aneurysm or surgical resection of the AVM if indicated.

## Intraparenchymal hemorrhage (IPH) (Fig. 4-8):

■ Etiologies: Hypertension, amyloid angiopathy, metastatic hemorrhage, hemorrhagic conversion from ischemic stroke, or coagulopathic state

■ Clinical characteristics: Headaches, focal deficits

■ Imaging characteristics (CT): Hyperdensity contained within brain parenchyma

■ Management: Reversal of underlying coagulopathy, blood pressure control, surgical drainage if large

## Subdural hematoma (Fig. 4-9):

■ A collection of blood beneath the dura mater

■ Etiology: Trauma especially in the elderly or nonaccidental trauma in children leading to ruptured bridging veins

■ Imaging characteristics: **Crescent**-shaped hyperdensity (acute) or hypodensity (chronic) lesion that hugs the brain but not in the sulci

■ Management: Blood pressure control, surgical drainage if large, and seizure prophylaxis

## Epidural hematoma (Fig. 4-10):

■ A collection of blood outside the dura mater

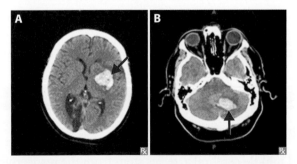

**FIGURE 4-8.** CT demonstrating (A) intraparenchymal hemorrhage in the left basal ganglia and (B) in the cerebellum.

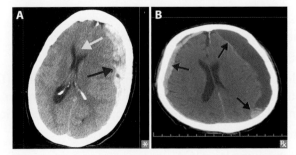

**FIGURE 4-9.** CT demonstrating (A) acute left subdural hematoma with midline shift and (B) acute on chronic subdural hematoma.

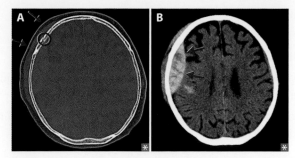

FIGURE 4-10. **CT demonstrating (A) skull fracture and (B) epidural hematoma.**

- Etiology: Trauma, injury to middle meningeal artery via blow to the pterion
- Clinical picture: Transient, lucid interval after head injury followed by a rapid deterioration
- Imaging characteristics: **Biconcave lens** shape that does not hug the cortex and does not cross suture lines
- Management: Blood pressure control, surgical drainage

## CEREBRAL VENOUS SINUS THROMBOSIS

- An occlusion in the cerebral venous sinus can lead to hemorrhage or infarct due to edema from poor drainage.
- Etiology: Hypercoagulable state (malignancy, oral contraceptive use, pregnancy, Factor V Leiden, antithrombin deficiency, Protein C & S deficiency, prothrombin gene mutation), dehydration trauma, or fracture.
- Clinical picture: Somnolence, headaches, papilledema, seizures, focal neurological deficits.
- Diagnostics: CT head without contrast, CT venogram head with contrast.
- Imaging characteristics: Hyperdensity (filling defect) on CT venogram, possible intraparenchymal hemorrhage, or hemorrhage in an atypical, nonarterial territory.
- Management: Anticoagulation is the mainstay of acute and subacute treatment.

## Clinical Syndromes

## ANTERIOR CIRCULATION

- Anterior and middle cerebral arteries stem from the respective internal carotid artery on each side.
- Anterior cerebral artery (ACA):
  - Anteromedial frontal lobe, caudate.
  - Contralateral leg weakness, urinary incontinence, abulia.
- Middle cerebral artery (MCA):
  - Clinical deficits depend on the proximity of the occlusion (the closer to the ICA, the more the deficits), and could involve the internal capsule, lateral geniculate nucleus (vision), motor and sensory cortices.
  - Contralateral motor weakness and sensory loss.
  - Aphasia if involving left MCA.
  - Left-sided hemineglect if involving right MCA (Fig. 4-11).

**KEY FACT**

Not all strokes manifest with contralateral deficits. Strokes that affect the brainstem could directly injure the ipsilateral cranial nuclei or nerve and therefore lead to ipsilateral symptoms.

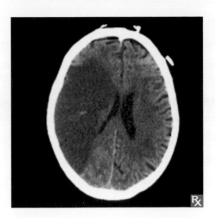

**FIGURE 4-11. CT head showing acute stroke in right MCA territory, from FA for USMLE1.**

## POSTERIOR CIRCULATION

- Vertebral arteries travel from or near the aorta and join to form the basilar artery which eventually bifurcates to the posterior cerebral arteries.
- Posterior cerebral artery (PCA):
  - Supplies the inferior temporal lobes, thalamus, and occipital lobes.
  - Occipital lobe infarct leads to contralateral homonymous hemianopsia (with macular sparing).
- Brainstem:
  - Crossed signs (body and face) since the ipsilateral cranial nerve nucleus is directly injured (ie, left face and right body affected).
  - Basilar perforators (lower midbrain or pons):
    - Lesions in the cortical spinal tract can lead to **Locked-in syndrome**: quadriplegia with preserved consciousness and vertical eye movements.
  - Anterior inferior cerebellar artery (lateral pons):
    - Lesions in the ipsilateral cranial nerve nuclei can lead to ipsilateral facial weakness or ipsilateral hearing loss, in addition to contralateral hemibody weakness.
  - Posterior inferior cerebellar artery (lateral medulla):
    - Lateral medullary syndrome/**Wallenberg syndrome:** Vertigo, nystagmus, nausea/vomiting, ipsilateral Horner syndrome, dysphagia, hoarseness, ipsilateral ataxia, loss of pain and temperature on contralateral body but ipsilateral face, and vertical diplopia.
  - Anterior spinal artery (medial medulla):
    - Contralateral weakness and proprioception deficit.
    - Ipsilateral tongue deviation.

## SECONDARY CAUSES OF STROKE

### CNS Vasculitis

- Autoimmune, inflammatory disease of medium- and small-caliber cerebral arteries in the absence of other systemic vasculitic manifestations.

  → Subacute presentation of headache and progressive/stepwise neurological deficits.
- Equal gender distribution, onset usually in 40s and 50s.
- May have nonspecific markers of inflammation such as elevated ESR.
- MRI shows nonspecific white matter disease and is rarely normal.

- Angiography may show "beading" of blood vessels.
- Brain and meningeal biopsy is gold standard but still only ~75% sensitive.
- CSF may have aseptic meningitis pattern, but may be normal.

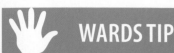

*Kernohan notch phenomenon (a false localizing sign): uncal herniation can cause compression of the contralateral cerebral peduncle, causing ipsilateral hemiparesis.*

## Common Patterns for Localization

- **Pure motor hemiplegia:** Internal capsule or ventral pontine stroke
- **Pure sensory stroke:** Lateral thalamic stroke
- **Clumsy hand–dysarthria:** Paramedian midpontine stroke
- **Ipsilateral hemiparesis–ataxia:** Pons, midbrain, or internal capsule stroke

## Herniation Syndromes

- **Subfalcine:** Displacement of the medial frontoparietal cortex under falx cerebri
  - Causes compression of the ACA, resulting in contralateral leg weakness and altered mental status (AMS)
- **Transtentorial:** Central, downward herniation that causes displacement of the brainstem
  - Caused by edema
  - Patients have AMS, loss of brainstem reflexes such as pupillary reflex, corneal reflex, oculocephalic reflex, gag or cough reflex, and posturing
- **Uncal:** Medial temporal lobe herniating downward
  - Causes a CN III palsy (blown pupil with down and out gaze)
- **Cerebellar tonsillar:** Displacement of cerebellar tonsils into foramen magnum
  - Causes compression of the medulla (respiratory arrest, posturing, Altered Mental Status (AMS), dysrhythmias)

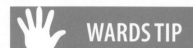

*Strokes of the cerebellum can cause rapid cerebellar herniation during peak edema window of 3-5 days.*

### MANAGEMENT OF ELEVATED ICP/HERNIATION SYNDROMES

Emergent airway, breathing, and circulation (ABCs): Secure airway, assess need for mechanical ventilation.

Treat the underlying cause: Surgical removal of space-occupying lesion.

- Hyperosmolar therapy: Mannitol bolus 0.5 to 1 g/kg IV, target serum osmolarity 300 to 310 mOsm/L (risk of acute tubular necrosis with serum osmolarity > 320); may → paradoxical worsening of midline shift secondary to greater efficacy on the side of brain with intact blood–brain barrier in patients with large strokes. Hypertonic IV saline such as 3% or 23.4% are also used to counter cerebral edema. Steroids (only for vasogenic edema; contraindicated in cytotoxic edema from brain trauma and stroke).
- Hyperventilation: Target $PCO_2$ to 28 to 32 mm Hg, rapidly reduces ICP through vasoconstriction → decreasing volume of intracranial blood, short-lived effect on ICP, slow normalization of respiratory rate on ventilator to avoid rebound effect.
- Ventricular CSF drainage with a goal ICP <20 mm $H_2O$. Lumbar drainage contraindicated in the setting of mass lesions or midline shift, but may be effective in cryptococcal meningitis or idiopathic intracranial hypertension.

**Case 1:** A 65-year-old man presents to the emergency department with difficulty with speech and weakness in the right upper extremity. He was last known to be neurologically normal 3 hours prior to presentation. He has a medical history of atrial fibrillation, hypertension, hyperlipidemia, and type 2 diabetes mellitus. He smokes approximately one pack of cigarettes daily for the past 12 years. Physical examination is notable for 2/5 power in the right upper extremity and word-finding difficulty. A noncontrast head CT is performed, which does not demonstrate an intracranial hemorrhage.

What is the treatment in this patient?

A. Aspirin
B. Intravenous tPA
C. 3% oxygen therapy
D. Hemispherectomy
E. Intravenous rituximab

The correct answer is B. This patient has multiple stroke risk factors and presents with findings consistent with left MCA stroke (aphasia and right-sided weakness). Intravenous tPA should be administered.

**Case 2:** A 58-year-old woman presents to the emergency room with a severe headache of sudden onset. Her symptoms began approximately 2 hours ago after she was at the gym lifting weights. She denies any head trauma, nausea, or vomiting. Physical examination is unremarkable. A CT head and neck without contrast is normal. An emergency lumbar puncture is done and demonstrates elevated red blood cells that do not diminish from tube 1 to 4. In the ER she describes it as the worst headache of her life.

What is the most likely diagnosis?

A. Subarachnoid hemorrhage
B. Migraine headache without aura
C. Carotid artery dissection
D. Cavernous sinus thrombosis
E. Giant cell arteritis

The correct answer is A. The signs and symptoms are consistent with subarachnoid hemorrhage.

**Case 3:** A 71-year-old woman presents to the emergency department after developing slurred speech approximately 2 hours ago. Once she arrived, her symptoms gradually resolved. CT head without contrast was unremarkable. CT angiogram of head and neck with contrast shows no significant stenosis intracranially while the left internal carotid artery had 50% to 69% stenosis after the bifurcation extracranially. MRI brain with diffusion-weighted sequences does not provide evidence of an infarct. Her blood pressure is 130/90. The most likely diagnosis is:

A. TIA
B. Multi-infarct dementia
C. Complex migraine with aura
D. Meningioma
E. Hypertensive encephalopathy

The correct answer is A. This patient has suffered a TIA likely due to her stenotic carotid ("symptomatic carotid"). Her symptoms have resolved and MRI showed no sign of infarction. She does not have other symptoms consistent with migraine, dementia, or meningioma. Her BP was only slightly elevated. The patient could be considered for carotid revascularization interventions such as endarterectomy or stenting to prevent future strokes.

# CHAPTER 5

# CNS INFECTIONS

In this chapter, we review the spectrum of central nervous system (CNS) infections in a systematic manner: Definition, Symptoms (including both history and exam), Microbiology, Differential Diagnosis, Work-up/Diagnostics, Treatment/Management, and then Prognosis/Complications.

## Brain Abscess

Brain abscesses commonly occur when bacteria or fungi infect part of the brain. As a result, swelling and irritation (inflammation) develop. Infected brain cells, white blood cells, live and dead bacteria or fungi collect in an area of the brain. Tissue forms around this area and creates a mass.

### Symptoms:

- The classic triad of symptoms for brain abscess is *fever, headache, and focal neurological symptoms*, but only a minority of patients develop all three.
- A brain abscess usually presents as an acute to subacute mass lesion.
- Symptoms of elevated intracranial pressure (ICP) include headache, nausea, and vomiting, which may worsen with the Valsalva maneuver or when the patient lies down.
- Seizures occur and are often generalized with a focal onset, but this may not be easily apparent by history or observation.

### Exam:

- Focal neurological signs are often absent or may be extremely subtle.
- Papilledema is frequently absent because the abscess evolves too rapidly for this sign to appear.

### Differential diagnosis:

- *Staphylococcus aureus:* Usually associated with a penetrating head wound, neurosurgical procedure, or bacterial endocarditis.
- *Streptococcus:* Often arises from sinusitis or dental infections.
- Gram-negative rods: Include *Haemophilus, Pseudomonas, Escherichia coli, Enterobacter;* often seen in neonates and the immunocompromised and with an associated meningitis.
- Other: *Aspergillus, Mucor:* Usually due to direct extension from the sinuses in patients who are immunocompromised or suffer from diabetes and is often fatal.

### Diagnosis:

- Brain magnetic resonance imaging (MRI) with contrast is the test of choice: Demonstrates ring-enhancing lesion; head CT with contrast can be used if MRI is not available but is not as sensitive.
- CSF exam is usually unhelpful, and LP may cause brain herniation and death; CSF exam is usually normal.

### Treatment:

- Broad antibiotic coverage should be initiated, usually with a third-generation cephalosporin and metronidazole.
- In the setting of a neurosurgical procedure or head trauma, vancomycin should be used to cover *Staphylococcus.* Coverage can be narrowed when speciation and sensitivities are available. Total duration of therapy is 4 to 8 weeks.

- Surgical aspiration or excision is often required.
- Supportive care, including control of surrounding edema and elevated ICP and seizures, is essential.

**Complications:**
Early diagnosis and initiation of appropriate antibiotic therapy dramatically reduces mortality.

- Acute complications include intraventricular rupture, which substantially worsens prognosis, hydrocephalus, and seizures.

**Prognosis:**
- Overall, 5% to 10% mortality rate.

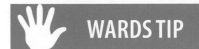

**WARDS TIP**

Antibiotics may be started up to several hours before CSF is obtained without affecting culture results.

## Spinal Epidural Abscess

Usually seen in patients with diabetes, back trauma, and IV drug abuse, who are immunocompromised, pregnant, and following back surgery.

**Symptoms:**
- Usually present acutely or subacutely and represent a neurological emergency.
- The initial symptom is usually a localized, severe pain on the back over the site of the abscess. This may be followed by radicular pain and then by myelopathic symptoms as the abscess compresses the spinal cord.
- Myelopathic symptoms include incoordination due to loss of position sense, gait ataxia, stiffness, and spasms in the legs due to impairment of the cortical spinal tract, numbness below a spinal level, and loss of bowel and bladder control.

**Exam:**
- Fever is helpful but is often not present or is attributed to other causes.
- The patient will usually have focal pain to percussion over the spine.
- Myelopathic signs include loss of position and vibration sense, upper motor neuron signs, and a spinal sensory level.

**Differential diagnosis:**
- *Staphylococcus aureus:* The most common etiological agent.
- *Staphylococcus epidermidis:* Associated with neurosurgical procedures.
- Tuberculosis: Can cause chronic epidural abscess and is associated with HIV infection and injection drug use.

**Diagnosis:**
- Spine MRI with contrast is the test of choice.
- CSF exam is usually unhelpful.
- Blood cultures are positive about half the time.

**Treatment:**
- Early diagnosis and treatment significantly reduce mortality.
- Almost always requires urgent open surgery for debridement.
- Broad antibiotic coverage should be initiated, usually with a third-generation cephalosporin and vancomycin.

- If gram-negative organisms are suspected, use gentamicin.
- Coverage can be narrowed when speciation and sensitivities are available.
- Total duration of therapy is 4 to 8 weeks, depending on clinical course and follow-up imaging.

**Prognosis:**

- Overall, 5% to 15% fatality rate; residual deficits depend on degree and duration of acute neurological deficit, degree of cord compression, and length of abscess.

## Meningitis

Inflammation or infection of the meninges, usually caused by bacteria, viruses, or fungi, but occasionally caused by other infectious agents or noninfectious conditions.

**Symptoms:**

- Depend on the etiology of the meningitis, but typically include fever, headache, and nuchal rigidity (neck stiffness).

**Exam:**

- Clinical signs include evidence of meningeal irritation, including nuchal rigidity, Kernig sign, and Brudzinski sign. Both of these signs occur because when the meninges are irritated, placing a stretch on them produces pain, causing the patient to take action to relieve that stretch.
- **Kernig sign:** Passive flexion of the patient's hip and extension of the knee causes the patient to flex his or her neck.
- **Brudzinski sign:** Passive flexion of the neck causes the patient to flex his or her legs.

**Diagnosis:**

- By definition, inflammation must be present, so spinal fluid examination will reveal a pleocytosis (increased cell count) (Table 5-1).
- Patients with meningitis may have elevated ICP; perform head CT prior to LP to assess the safety of the procedure.

**TABLE 5-1. CSF Profiles in Meningitis**

| | Normal Values | Bacterial | Viral | Fungal |
|---|---|---|---|---|
| Opening pressure (mm Hg) | 50–80 | Elevated (100–300) | Normal or slightly elevated (80–100) | Elevated |
| Pleocytosis (WBCs/mm³) | 0–5 | Usually >1000 | Usually >100 | Usually >100 |
| % Neutrophils | 0 | >50% | <20% | Variable |
| Protein (mg/dL) | 20–45 | Usually >100 | Usually >45 | Variable |
| Glucose (mg/dL) | Two-thirds of serum glucose | ↓ | Normal | Often very ↓ |
| Other tests | | Gram stain and culture | Viral polymerase chain reaction (PCR) | India ink, culture, cryptococcal antigen |

Reproduced with permission from Rafii M. *First Aid for the Neurology Boards, 2nd ed.* New York: McGraw Hill; 2015.

**Differential diagnosis:**

■ Systemic infection or sepsis; trauma or closed head injury or child abuse; multiple metabolic abnormalities (hypoglycemia, ketoacidosis, electrolyte imbalance, uremia, toxic exposure); seizure; brain tumor; subarachnoid or intracranial hemorrhage; epidural abscess.

## BACTERIAL MENINGITIS

**Symptoms:**

■ Typically include fever, headache, photophobia, nausea, vomiting, irritability, and lethargy, proceeding to further clouding of consciousness and, ultimately, death.

■ The course is frequently fulminant, with rapid neurologic deterioration; therefore, initiation of appropriate antibiotic treatment must not be delayed (Table 5-2).

**Exam:**

■ Evidence of meningeal irritation, though this can be lacking in children, the elderly, and the deeply comatose.

■ Fever may be ≥103°F or higher.

■ Focal neurological signs may also appear.

**Differential diagnosis:**

There are several different bacteria that can cause meningitis in various demographic groups. See below for details.

**Diagnosis:**

■ CSF exam showing a predominantly neutrophilic pleocytosis is strongly suggestive; should prompt broad-coverage antibiotic treatment; however, in the proper clinical setting, do not delay treatment in order to obtain CSF.

■ Because many types of bacteria can cause enough brain edema to make an LP hazardous, consider brain imaging prior to CSF exam.

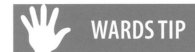

**WARDS TIP**

When bacterial meningitis is suspected, antibiotic treatment must be initiated emergently, even without identification of the causative organism. Treatment is usually directed primarily against *S. pneumoniae* and *N. meningitidis*, the most common causes of community-acquired meningitis.

| TABLE 5-2. Common Causes of Bacterial Meningitis | |
|---|---|
| **Age** | **Bacteria** |
| Neonates (<1-year-old), due to exposure in the birth canal | Group B streptococci and gram-negative enteric bacilli, particularly *Escherichia coli* |
| Children ≥1-year-old and adults | *Streptococcus pneumoniae* and *Neisseria meningitidis* |
| Older adults (>50-year-old) | *S. pneumoniae* and gram-negative bacilli, including *Haemophilus influenza, E. coli, Enterobacter, and Pseudomonas* |
| Recurrent meningitis, CSF leak, head trauma, due to skin and nasopharyngeal colonization | *S. pneumoniae* and nontypeable *H. influenza* |
| Pneumonia (adults 18-50 years old) | *S. pneumoniae* |
| Chronic lung disease | *Pseudomonas* |
| Chronic urinary tract infection | *E. coli* or *Enterobacter* |
| Sinusitis, otitis media | Nontypeable *H. influenza, S. pneumoniae* |
| Immunosuppressed and/or elderly | *Listeria monocytogenes* |
| Neurosurgical patients | *S. pneumoniae*, nontypeable *H. influenza*, and *S. aureus* |

Reproduced with permission from Rafii M. *First Aid for the Neurology Boards, 2nd ed.* New York: McGraw Hill; 2015

## KEY FACT

CSF exam showing predominantly neutrophils is strongly suggestive of bacterial meningitis; should prompt broad-coverage antibiotic treatment; however, do not delay treatment in order to obtain CSF.

**Treatment:**

- Based on the specific bacteria involved and their sensitivity to antibiotics. There should be no delay in starting antibiotics for presumed meningitis.
- Typically, broad-spectrum antibiotics are given empirically (based on clinical judgment) and adjusted based on sensitivities from CSF. They can be discontinued once bacterial meningitis is ruled out.

## MENINGOCOCCAL MENINGITIS

- Caused by a gram-negative diplococcus, *Neisseria meningitidis*.
- Typically associated with a rash, which can vary from petechial to purpuric. Such a rash, together with fever and hypotension/shock, is strong evidence for this type of infection.
- Bacterial antigen can be detected from CSF.
- **Waterhouse-Friderichsen** syndrome (**hemorrhagic adrenalitis**): disease of the adrenal glands most commonly caused by the bacterium *Neisseria meningitidis* resulting in massive hemorrhage into one or (usually) both adrenal glands.
- Characterized by overwhelming bacterial infection meningococcemia, low blood pressure and shock, disseminated intravascular coagulation (DIC) with widespread purpura, and rapidly developing adrenocortical insufficiency.

## PNEUMOCOCCAL MENINGITIS

- Caused by *Streptococcus pneumoniae,* gram-positive cocci.
- Leading cause of bacterial meningitis worldwide.
- Often, a history of productive cough, dyspnea, and constitutional symptoms in the days prior to onset of meningitis-like symptoms. Concomitant pneumonia is common. Pneumonia is often associated with bacteremia and, therefore, with meningitis.
- *S. pneumoniae* is also a common cause of otitis media and acute sinusitis, which can provide a source of meningitis, by either hematogenous spread or direct extension.

## HAEMOPHILUS MENINGITIS

- Caused by gram-negative coccobacilli.
- Frequent history of an upper respiratory tract infection preceding onset of meningitis, with hematogenous spread.
- Hib is an encapsulated organism, so patients with splenectomy (functional or surgical) are at increased risk.

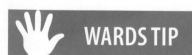

## WARDS TIP

Four tubes are usually drawn during a lumbar puncture, an increase in RBC from tube 1 to tube 4 usually indicates an intracranial bleed (subarachnoid hemorrhage) if the tap is non-traumatic.

## TUBERCULOUS MENINGITIS

- Caused by the acid-fast bacillus (AFB) *Mycobacterium tuberculosis*.
- Common in developing countries.
- Basilar meningitis can occur with cranial neuropathies.
- TB is often seen in association with HIV, malnourishment, alcoholism, and crowded living conditions such as jails and homeless shelters.

- Often preceded by weeks of general malaise and other nonspecific constitutional symptoms.
- CSF pleocytosis is often lymphocytic, protein is elevated, and glucose is extremely low.
- Chest x-ray may show evidence of pulmonary TB, and diagnosis may be made by sputum AFB smear.
- CSF AFB smear and culture are frequently negative, or may take weeks to grow.

**Treatment:**
- Optimal treatment regimen is isoniazid, rifampin, pyrazinamide, ethambutol, and streptomycin.

**Complications:**
- Early diagnosis and initiation of appropriate antibiotic therapy dramatically reduces mortality and morbidity.
- Acute complications include hemorrhagic stroke, cerebritis, ventriculitis, abscess, hydrocephalus, and seizures.
- Permanent neurological sequelae include behavioral and developmental difficulties, hearing loss, seizures, motor deficits, and ataxia.

**Prognosis:**
- Overall, 20% to 25% fatality rate.

# FUNGAL MENINGITIS

- Can present with an acute or chronic course.
- Most patients will be immunocompromised, usually by HIV infection, malignancy, posttransplant immunosuppression, diabetes, or steroid use.

**Differential diagnosis:**
- *Cryptococcus:* See below.
- *Coccidioides:* Found in southwestern United States, Mexico, Central and South America; exposure to soil dust (construction, farmers); CSF pleocytosis will often include an eosinophilia.
- *Histoplasma:* Found in Mississippi and Ohio river valleys; exposure to bat and bird droppings (exploring caves, cleaning chicken coops).
- *Blastomyces:* Found in same areas as *Histoplasma* but also in upper Midwest and Great Lakes regions.
- *Candida:* Seen in premature neonates possibly related to vaginal yeast infection of mother.

**Diagnosis:**
- Depends on the fungus.
- Many **fungi** can also be observed with **India ink** staining of the CSF.
- Antigen and/or antibody testing can be used for some.

**Treatment:**
- Depends on the sensitivities of the particular infecting organism: Amphotericin B, fluconazole, itraconazole, voriconazole, caspofungin.
- Empiric antifungal therapy (usually with amphotericin B) is sometimes reasonable in high-risk patients who are severely ill with meningitis, but without an identified organism.

**WARDS TIP**

Severe diffuse headache and obstructive hydrocephalus are often seen in patients with fungal meningitis.

**Prognosis:**

- Prior to the development of amphotericin B, most fungal infections of the nervous system were fatal.

## CRYPTOCOCCAL MENINGITIS

- Most common CNS fungal infection
- Usually occurs in immunocompromised patients

**Symptoms:**

- Chronic meningitis and altered mental status. Increased ICP is very common as fungus blocks CSF flow.

**Diagnosis**: CSF—India-ink, positive, Crypto Antigen positive.

**Treatment**: Amphotericin B or fluconazole.

## CNS Toxoplasmosis

- Infection caused by *Toxoplasma gondii,* a small intracellular parasite.
- Occurs with CD4 counts <100. Congenital forms also occur, usually causing periventricular calcification.

**Symptoms/Exam:**

- Focal neurological deficits and mental status changes.

**Differential diagnosis:**

- The biggest consideration is CNS lymphoma.
- Frequently, patients with a compatible presentation are treated for toxoplasmosis, and if there is no improvement within 2 weeks, strong consideration is given to a lymphoma diagnosis.

**Diagnosis:**

- Brain MRI with contrast typically demonstrates *multifocal* ring-enhancing lesions, although can be unifocal.
- *Toxoplasma* serologies may help differentiate CNS toxoplasmosis from CNS lymphoma.

**Treatment:**

- Pyrimethamine, sulfadiazine, and folinic acid.

**Prognosis:**

- Rapid response to proper treatment.

## Viral Diseases

## HERPES ENCEPHALITIS

- Caused by herpes simplex virus type 1, except in neonates where it is associated with maternal genital HSV type 2.

**Symptoms:**

- Presents, as with any encephalopathy or encephalitis, with mental status and behavioral changes.
- Often a prodromal viral-like illness including fever, general malaise, headache, neck stiffness.
- Because organism has predisposition to temporal lobes, patients can have profound memory loss and seizures.
- There may be olfactory and gustatory hallucinations.

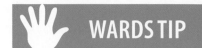

**WARDS TIP**

Behavioral and personality change, followed by complex partial seizures, is often seen in HSV encephalitis.

**Exam:**

- Focal neurological signs including motor signs and cranial neuropathies.

**Diagnosis:**

- CSF examination: Since this infection causes hemorrhagic encephalitis, the presence of non-clearing red blood cells strongly suggests the diagnosis in the proper clinical setting.
- HSV PCR of CSF has high sensitivity and specificity and is thus the diagnostic test of choice.
- Brain MRI will typically show T2 bright changes and edema in temporal, cingulate, and orbitofrontal lobes.
- Electroencephalogram (EEG) may show temporal spikes.

**Treatment:**

- Intravenous acyclovir should be started immediately in any patient with a compatible clinical presentation and continued for 14-21 days if diagnosis confirmed.

**Complications:**

- Survivors frequently have severe problems with forming new memories, persistent cognitive deficits, and seizures.

**Prognosis:**

- Fifty percent severe morbidity or mortality, especially if treatment is delayed.

## WEST NILE ENCEPHALITIS

**Symptoms/Exam:**

- Presents, as with any encephalopathy or encephalitis, with mental status and behavioral changes.
- Often a prodromal viral-like illness including fever, general malaise, headache, neck stiffness.
- West Nile can also cause a flaccid paralysis, similar to poliomyelitis.

**Diagnosis:**

- Positive West Nile serology and a compatible clinical presentation.
- CSF examination: Nonspecific lymphocytic pleocytosis.

**Treatment:**

- Supportive.

**Prognosis:**

■ Mortality low, but persistent deficits common.

## POLIOMYELITIS

■ Infection of lower motor neurons by an enterovirus, transmitted by fecal-oral route.
■ Extremely rare in the United States because of widespread use of polio vaccine, but historically was common cause of paralysis of one or more extremities, and still occurs in underdeveloped countries.

**Symptoms:**

■ Mild flulike illness; myalgias; aseptic meningitis, which usually resolves with no further problems.
■ Paralytic poliomyelitis: Rapid limb and bulbar weakness, most patients recover completely, but some have residual weakness and atrophy of one or more extremities.

**Diagnosis:** Serological testing, viral isolation from stool; virus is rarely if ever isolated from CSF.

**Treatment:** Supportive/symptomatic only.

## RABIES

■ Caused by rhabdovirus.

**Symptoms/Exam:**

■ Transmitted by bite of rabid animal, most commonly a bat, but found in any mammal, including dogs, raccoons, and skunks.
■ There is prolonged incubation period, usually 20 to 60 days, from time of bite to onset of rabies symptoms. During this time, virus spreads along peripheral nerves from site of inoculation to the CNS. Prodromal symptoms last a few days and include fever, chills, malaise, fatigue, insomnia, anorexia, headache, anxiety, and irritability.
■ About one-half develop pain, paresthesias, or pruritus at or close to bite site, which may reflect infection of the dorsal root ganglia.
■ Encephalitic rabies affects about 80%. This is the classic/stereotypical form, in which patients have episodes of hyperexcitability alternating with periods of relative lucidity. They may have aggressive behavior, confusion, hallucinations, and seizures.
■ Autonomic dysfunction is common and includes hypersalivation, sweating, and piloerection.
■ The disease progresses through paralysis, coma, multisystem organ failure, and death.

**Differential diagnosis:**

■ Often misdiagnosed as psychiatric or laryngopharyngeal disorder.
■ Rabies has been misdiagnosed as Creutzfeldt-Jakob disease (CJD).
■ Tetanus can cause laryngospasm along with spasm and rigidity of diffuse muscles, but usually not associated with encephalopathy.

**KEY FACT**

The rabies virus replicates in muscle and binds to the nicotinic acetylcholine receptor. It can lead to pralaysis including respiratory failure.

**Diagnosis:**

- Rabies viral RNA can be detected by PCR from brain, saliva, and CSF.

**Treatment:**

- After clinical symptoms emerge, supportive only.
- Postexposure prophylaxis (PEP) can prevent onset of clinical rabies and subsequent death. PEP includes both active and passive immunization.

**Prognosis:**

- Uniformly fatal after symptom onset.

## VARICELLA ZOSTER VIRUS (VZV)

- Also known as "shingles."

**Symptoms:**

- Vesicular rash in a dermatomal pattern, usually on one side of body along the course of one or more cutaneous nerves.
- Frequently painful or pruritic, rash may follow onset of pain by a few days.
- Spontaneous reactivation of latent varicella zoster virus (VZV), which, after an initial infection usually as a child (chickenpox), lies dormant in dorsal root ganglia of spinal nerves or fifth cranial nerve.

**Incidence:** Increases with age and immunosuppression.

**Diagnosis:** Usually clinical, but can do **Tzanck** prep from a vesicle, which will show **multinucleated giant cells**.

**Complications:**

- Ophthalmic zoster can result in blindness.
- Post-herpetic neuralgia can last months to years after shingles and cause significant distress.

**Treatment:** Acyclovir, valacyclovir, or famciclovir, started as soon as possible and no later than 3 days after onset of rash. It shortens the duration of illness and decreases incidence of post-herpetic neuralgia.

## RAMSAY-HUNT SYNDROME

Shingles involving the facial nerve with triad of ipsilateral facial paralysis, otalgia, and vesicles near the ear and auditory canal, often with tinnitus and vertigo. Deafness may occur.

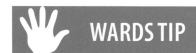 **WARDS TIP**

Gabapentin is often used for post-herpetic neuralgia from shingles.

## Neuro-Lyme Disease

- *Borrelia burgdorferi* transmitted by bite of Ixodes tick, also known as deer tick.
- Ixodes ticks and Borrelia burgdorferi are found in the Northeast, mid-Atlantic, and upper Midwest, and not in the Southwest.
- Transmission usually occurs in late spring or summer.

**Symptoms/Exam:**

- Lyme disease causes a wide variety of symptoms. Erythema migrans rash occurs at time of initial infection, looks like a bull's eye, with a pale center, surrounded by a red ring. Rash expands in diameter over several days before resolving.

- Migratory myalgias, arthralgias, fatigue, and general malaise common.
- Most common neurological involvement is **facial palsy**, sometimes bilaterally. Other cranial nerve palsies may also be seen.
- Headache and aseptic meningitis are also common.

### Diagnosis:

- As with any condition, history trumps all else, and description of appropriate rash, together with exposure to a tick environment, should prompt treatment. However, many patients are concerned about Lyme disease, and will describe a rash that may not be typical of erythema migrans. Patients also may not see the rash.

### Treatment:

- Oral doxycycline is effective for non-neurological Lyme disease and probably for Lyme meningitis and facial nerve palsies; IV ceftriaxone is needed for more severe CNS involvement.
- The most common cause of apparent antibiotic failure in Lyme disease is misdiagnosis.
- Prevention includes use of insect repellant with DEET and careful examination and washing of body after exposure to tick environment, because transmission requires >24 hours of tick attachment.

### Complications:

- Following confirmed and appropriately treated Lyme disease, some patients develop a poorly defined syndrome of subjective complaints, including depression, memory and concentration problems, myalgias, and fatigue.

## Bell's Palsy

- Bell's palsy is a peripheral palsy of the facial nerve that results in muscle weakness on one side of the face (Fig. 5-1).
- Affected patients develop unilateral facial paralysis over one to three days with forehead involvement and no other neurologic abnormalities.
- Symptoms typically peak in the first week and then gradually resolve over three weeks to three months.
- Bell's palsy is more common in patients with diabetes, and although it can affect persons of any age, incidence peaks in the 40s.
- Bell's palsy has been traditionally defined as idiopathic; however, one possible etiology is infection with herpes simplex virus type 1. A broad differential diagnosis must be considered (Table 5-3).
- Laboratory evaluation, when indicated by history or risk factors, may include testing for diabetes mellitus and Lyme disease.
- A common short-term complication of Bell's palsy is incomplete eyelid closure with resultant dry eye and corneal abrasion.
- A less common long-term complication is permanent facial weakness with muscle contractures.

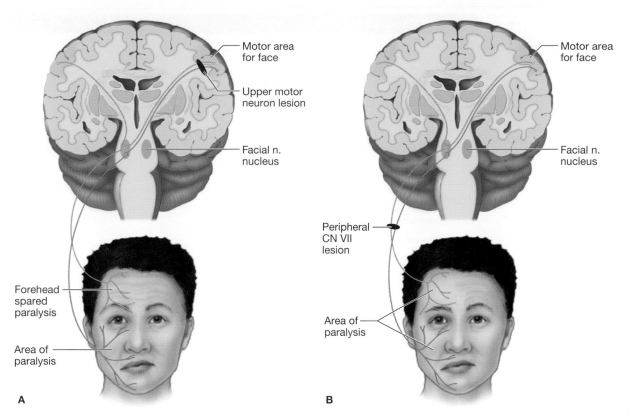

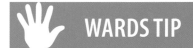

**FIGURE 5-1. Patients with (A) a facial nerve lesion and (B) a supranuclear lesion with forehead sparing.** Reproduced with permission from Kevin J. Knoop, Lawrence B. Stack, R. Jason Thurman, Alan B. Storrow. *The Atlas of Emergency Medicine, 5e.* New York: McGraw Hill; 2020.

■ Approximately 70% to 80% of patients will recover spontaneously; however, treatment with a seven-day course of acyclovir or valacyclovir and a tapering course of prednisone, initiated within three days of the onset of symptoms, is recommended to reduce the time to full recovery and increase the likelihood of complete recuperation.

**WARDS TIP**

Forehead is affected in Peripheral CN7 palsy, Forehead is spared in Central CN7 palsy.

## Neurosyphilis

Treponema pallidum is sexually transmitted and causes a wide variety of symptoms.

**Symptoms/Exam:**

■ Neurological involvement occurs during tertiary syphilis, usually months to years after initial infection; often asymptomatic.

■ Chronic meningitis is the most common neurological manifestation, in up to 25% of cases.

■ Focal symptoms and signs may occur due to granuloma, or "gumma," formation.

■ Stroke may occur secondary to vasculitic involvement.

■ **Tabes dorsalis** refers to involvement of dorsal columns with loss of proprioception and vibration sensation, which can lead to severe gait disturbance and/or incoordination. **Argyll Robertson** pupil may be seen (irregular, small pupil that accommodates but does not respond to light).

| TABLE 5-3. Causes of Bell Palsy |
| --- |
| Idiopathic |
| Pregnancy |
| Guillain-Barré syndrome |
| Lyme disease (may present as bifacial weakness) |
| Herpes zoster (Ramsay Hunt syndrome) |
| Neoplasms |
| Sarcoidosis |
| Head trauma |
| Acute intermittent porphyria |
| Lead poisoning |
| Brainstem infarction (rare) |

Source: Reproduced with permission from Halter JB, Ouslander JG, Studenski S, et al. *Hazzard's Geriatric Medicine and Gerontology, 7e.* New York: McGraw Hill; 2017.

### Diagnosis:

- CSF exam demonstrates lymphocytic pleocytosis (usually mild), elevated protein, and positive Venereal Disease Research Laboratory (VDRL) test.
- Serum VDRL and rapid plasma reagin (RPR) are nontreponemal tests that are nonspecific, but useful for screening. Fluorescent treponemal antibody absorption test (FTA-ABS) is specific treponemal antibody test used to confirm positive VDRL or RPR.
- CSF VDRL is specific but not sensitive for neurosyphilis.
- Positive serum FTA-ABS and positive CSF VDRL is sufficient to diagnose neurosyphilis. A patient with positive serology and neurological signs and symptoms should be treated for presumed neurosyphilis, especially if there is a CSF pleocytosis, even if CSF VDRL is negative.

### Treatment:

- Penicillin G 4 million units IV q4h for 10 to 14 days.
- Monitor CSF at 6 weeks, 3, 6, 12, and 24 months. VDRL titer should ↓ at least fourfold within 9 months of treatment.

## Neurocysticercosis

- Infection usually caused by ingestion of the parasite *Taenia solium,* a pork tapeworm.
- Endemic to Central and South America and being seen with ↑ frequency in the United States among immigrants from that part of the world.

**Symptoms:** Extremely common cause of seizures worldwide.

**Diagnosis:** Brain imaging reveals multiple calcified cysts.

**Treatment:** Albendazole or praziquantel, sometimes with steroids; anticonvulsants as needed.

## Progressive Multifocal Leukoencephalopathy

**Cause:** Reactivation of latent JC virus. CD4 counts <200. Can also occur in cancer patients (especially leukemia and lymphoma), and in patients who have been immunosuppressed for organ transplants. Rare side effect with using natalizumab for multiple sclerosis.

**Symptoms:**

- Personality change
- Cognitive decline
- Hemiparesis or hemisensory deficits
- Visual field cuts or cortical blindness
- Aphasias
- Cerebellar symptoms

**Diagnosis:** Brain MRI reveals multifocal, nonenhancing white matter lesions (begins occipitally).

**Treatment:** Cytarabine 2 mg/kg per day for 5 days each month.

**Prognosis:** 80% die in 9 months.

**Case 1:** A 29-year-old man presents to the emergency department with a headache. His headache was initially mild but then subsequently worsened over the course of 48 hours. He reports fevers, chills, photophobia, and neck stiffness. He denies any recent respiratory illness. His temperature is 101°F (38.3°C), blood pressure is 118/77 mm Hg, pulse is 112/min, and respirations are 23/min. Physical examination is notable for nuchal rigidity and petechial hemorrhages in the skin. An emergent lumbar puncture is performed, which demonstrates high WBC (neutrophil predominant) and low glucose.

What is the likely etiology of his symptoms?

A. Meningococcal meningitis
B. Neurocysticercosis
C. HSV encephalitis
D. Fungal meningitis
E. Spinal epidural abscess

The correct answer is A. This patient has meningococcal meningitis. High fever with headache and nuchal rigidity are consistent with meningitis. The absence of respiratory illness makes pneumococcal meningitis unlikely. Petechial hemorrhages are consistent with Neisseria meningitis as is the CSF profile.

**Case 2:** A 30-year-old male visiting from Brazil had a seizure while at church. In the emergency department, he is noted to be confused but slowly improving. He denies any seizures in the past and has no recent head injury or other illnesses. He denies drug abuse. CT shows multiple calcified cysts throughout the brain parenchyma.

The most appropriate treatment is:

A. Praziquantel
B. Sumatriptan
C. Valproic Acid
D. Colchicine
E. Gabapentin

The correct answer is A. Treatment for neurocysticercosis is praziquantel. This will treat the underlying cause of his seizure and hopefully prevent any future recurrence.

**Case 3:** A 73-year-old man presents with right facial paralysis, right ear pain, and vesicles near the right ear and auditory canal. He reports the vesicles erupted over the past 3 days and has also been experiencing mild tinnitus and vertigo. He denies any headache, nausea, or vomiting. His neurological exam is nonfocal.

What is the etiology of his diagnosis?

A. Herpes Virus type 2
B. Varicella Zoster Virus
C. Human Immunodeficiency virus
D. Toxoplasmosis
E. CNS lymphoma

The correct answer is B. The patient is suffering from Ramsay-Hunt syndrome which is caused by varicella zoster virus becoming reactivated in someone who had chicken pox earlier in life.

# CHAPTER 6

# DELIRIUM AND
# DEMENTIAS

In this chapter, we focus on the main symptoms and causes of delirium, and how to do the workup and management. Delirium is extremely common in the general inpatient setting and a frequent reason for neurology consultation. We also discuss dementia and its features as well as some of the most important types of dementia, their etiology, workup, and management. It will be important to be able to differentiate delirium versus dementia on the wards and on the exam.

## Delirium

### DEFINITION

Delirium has key symptoms that include inattention and a nonfocal exam, fluctuating activity level, altered consciousness. It is considered a medical emergency and can usually be resolved with control of primary etiology. It is often caused by

- Hypoxemia or metabolic derangements that lead to poor cerebral metabolism
- Poor/delayed neurotransmitter balance and homeostasis
- Drug effects on the central nervous system (CNS)
- Inflammation that could increase cytokines in the brain

### ETIOLOGY

General approach is to identify reversible causes such as infection and metabolic derangement, or iatrogenic causes such as polypharmacy, and rule out CNS etiologies.

- Stroke, seizure, meningitis, autoimmune encephalitis, traumatic brain injury, hypertensive encephalopathy, intracranial hypertension
- Infection, metabolic derangement:
  - Sepsis, hypoglycemia, adrenal insufficiency, diabetic ketoacidosis (DKA), hypothyroidism, vitamin deficiencies, symptomatic anemia
  - Common vitamin deficiencies:
    - Cobalamin (B12), thiamine (B1), folate (B9)
  - Immunocompromised state or infection:
    - HIV, syphilis, possibly HSV
- Organ failure:
  - Acute kidney injury, uremia, transaminitis, hyperammonemia, pancreatic insufficiency
  - Hyperammonemia theoretically but the serum level can be inconsistent
- Perioperative:
  - Recent surgery, anesthesia, blood loss, hypoxia
- Medication-induced or iatrogenic:
  - Anticholinergics, benzodiazepines, narcotics, antipsychotics, anti-Parkinson's disease medications
  - Polypharmacy: classically with several antiepileptic drugs
  - Adverse effects: chemotherapy, brain radiation

---

### WARDS TIP

A nonfocal exam refers to a neurological examination that does not reveal a specific locality to cognitive, motor, or sensory findings (eg, an infarct to the thalamus causing both sensory findings and some change in behavior). Descriptions like drowsiness or lethargy and altered consciousness are consistent with delirium.

### WARDS TIP

Consider medications, especially sedatives and anxiolytics. Ask about a patient's sleep pattern, especially how often vitals are collected overnight (interrupts their sleep!), metabolic panel, especially sodium and glucose (both hypo- and hyperglycemia), and if there is a reason for infection (eg, cough/SOB & URI or a foley & UTI).

### WARDS TIP

In dementia, the forest trail has fallen trees preventing one from passing through. A person may have moments of clarity, but specific cognitive path(way)s are inaccessible. In delirium, there is a dense fog throughout the forest. The path(way)s are accessible but difficult to find.

- Substance abuse:
  - Cocaine, amphetamine, heroin, alcohol intoxication, or alcohol withdrawal
- Toxins:
  - Carbon monoxide, organophosphates, botulinum
- Psychiatric conditions:
  - Hypomania, schizophrenia, delusions

## EVALUATION

- Check these standard labs for reversible causes:
  - Complete blood count
  - Comprehensive metabolic panel
  - Urinalysis
  - Urine toxicology screen panel
  - Chest X-ray
  - Electrocardiogram
  - HIV, RPR
  - Vitamin levels: B12, B1, B9
- Consider CT head and arterial or venous blood gas to rule out life-threatening conditions.
- Consider electroencephalogram (EEG) to rule out subclinical seizures if suspicion is high.
  - EEG findings for delirium often reveal diffuse slowing.

## MANAGEMENT

- Prevention:
  - Sleep hygiene and environmental optimization (ensure sunlight during day and prevent daytime sleep).
  - Monitor for underlying dementia symptoms that may be exacerbated in the hospital.
  - Limit pharmacologic factors (anticholinergics, benzos especially in elderly).
- Acute management of agitation:
  - Haloperidol IV or IM for those who can harm self or others, may need restraints for safety after attempts of reorientation. Watch out for extrapyramidal symptoms for first-generation antipsychotics.
  - Benzodiazepines for alcohol withdrawal (delirium tremens).
  - Avoid physical restraints especially in the elderly.

## Cerebral Edema

Acute hyponatremia or hypernatremia can cause brain damage. Correcting chronic hyponatremia or hypernatremia can also cause injury aggressively.

- Rapidly falling plasma sodium concentration causes *cerebral edema*.
- Rapidly rising concentration causes *osmotic demyelination*.
- *Rate of sodium correction depends on acuity and severity of symptoms.*

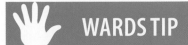

### WARDS TIP

The idea of poor brain reserve: Patients with underlying neuro-cognitive comorbidities such as dementia, multiple sclerosis, Parkinson's disease, or epilepsy have a lower threshold of having delirium when there is a toxo-metabolic insult or derangement because at baseline they now have less healthy brain to compensate.

### KEY FACT

**Alcohol intoxication:**
Acute consumption increases serotonin, dopamine, and GABA transmission, leading to variable behavioral changes. Give high-dose intravenous thiamine before giving glucose to prevent Wernicke encephalopathy.

Wernicke encephalopathy has the triad of delirium, ophthalmoplegia, and ataxia.

### KEY FACT

**Alcohol withdrawal:**
Early: Mild anxiety, labile emotions, confusion, fatigue, nausea.

12 to 48 hours from last drink: Withdrawal seizures (usually general tonic-clonic), and requires benzodiazepines or phenobarbital.

72 to 96 hours from last drink: *Delirium Tremens (DT)* – delirium ± psychomotor symptoms.

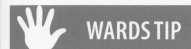

**WARDS TIP**

The rate of rise in the serum sodium concentration should be kept *below 10 mmol/L* during any 24-hour period. Treatment is supportive.

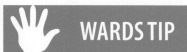

**WARDS TIP**

Symptoms of alcohol withdrawal/ delirium tremens—**HITS**
**H**allucinosis
**I**ncreased vitals (temp, BP, HR)/ Insomnia
**T**remors
**S**hakes/Seizures/Sweats/Stomach (nausea/vomiting)

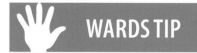

**WARDS TIP**

Avoid giving benzodiazepines or anticholinergics to the elderly as it can precipitate delirium.

**KEY FACT**

Delirious patients often lack medical decision-making capacity.

# Central Pontine Myelinolysis (Osmotic Demyelination Syndrome)

Central pontine myelinolysis (CPM) is a neurological disorder that most frequently occurs after too rapid medical correction of sodium deficiency (hyponatremia). The rapid rise in sodium concentration is accompanied by the movement of small molecules and pulls water from brain cells. Through a mechanism that is only partly understood, the shift in water and brain molecules leads to the destruction of myelin of the white matter of the CNS.

The initial symptoms of myelinolysis, which begin to appear 2 to 3 days after hyponatremia is corrected, include a depressed level of awareness, difficulty speaking (dysarthria or mutism), and difficulty swallowing (dysphagia). Additional symptoms often arise over the next 1 to 2 weeks, including impaired thinking, weakness or paralysis in the arms and legs, stiffness, impaired sensation, and difficulty with coordination.

# Dementia

Dementia is diagnosed when there are cognitive or behavioral (neuropsychiatric) symptoms that:

- Interfere with the ability to function at work or at usual activities.
- Represent a decline from previous levels of functioning and performing.
- Are not explained by delirium or major psychiatric disorder.

**Core Clinical Criteria for Dementia (National Institute on Aging-Alzheimer's Association [NIA-AA]):**

- At bedside measured using MOCA; in outpatient setting, perform neuropsychological testing as well.
  - Normal individuals are allowed a score of 26-30.
  - Score of 19-25 = Mild Cognitive Impairment (MCI).
  - Score of 11-21 = Mild Alzheimer's Disease (AD).
- Dementia involves impairment in at least two of four of the following domains which result in impairment in functionality at work/usual activities. This impairment is *not otherwise explained by delirium or a major psychiatric disorder.*
  - Impaired ability to acquire and remember new information.
    - Repetitive questions and conversations
    - Misplacing personal belongings
    - Forgetting events and appointments
    - Getting lost on familiar route
  - Impaired reasoning and handling of complex tasks; poor judgment.
    - Poor understanding of safety risks
    - Inability to manage finances
    - Poor decision-making
    - Inability to plan complex or sequential activities
  - Impaired visuospatial abilities.
    - Inability to recognize faces or common objects despite sufficient visual acuity

- – Inability to operate simple implements
- – Cannot orient clothing to body
- Impaired language functions (speaking, reading, writing).
  - – Difficulty thinking of common words while speaking; speaking with hesitations
  - – Speech, spelling, and writing errors
- Changes in personality, behavior, or comportment.
  - – Uncharacteristic mood fluctuations (ie, agitation)
  - – Impaired motivation, initiative, apathy, loss of drive, social withdrawal, decreased interest in previous activities, loss of empathy, compulsive or obsessive behaviors
  - – Socially unacceptable behaviors

## MILD COGNITIVE IMPAIRMENT (MCI)

- A decline in cognitive function with *preservation of most activities of daily living*, but NOT meeting criteria for dementia.
- Amnestic and nonamnestic variants:
  - Amnestic MCI is often due to underlying AD in pathology and can progress to AD.
- Early detection is essential to delaying progression.
  - 12% to 15% of nondemented patients >65 years old have MCI, with incidence of 1% per year.
  - 10% to 15% of MCI patients typically progress to dementia per year; 60% are demented at 5 years.
  - Severity of symptoms predicts rate of progression.
    - – Degree of memory impairment or multiple-domain MCI progress more rapidly.
  - Hippocampal atrophy on magnetic resonance imaging (MRI) predicts progression.

### Clinical diagnostic criteria:

- Concern regarding a change in cognition (history obtained from patient/informant/clinician/family)
- Impairment in one or more cognitive domains *for age and education:*
  - Memory
  - Executive function
  - Attention
  - Language
  - Visuospatial skills
- Preservation of independence in functional abilities
- Not demented (ie, the impairment should be so mild that the patient has no evidence of significant social or occupational functioning deficits)

### Pathophysiology:

- The pathophysiology of amnestic MCI is often due to underlying AD. In this case it is referred to as Prodromal AD.
  - Similar to AD—medial temporal lobe atrophy and intracellular neurofibrillary tangles consisting of phosphorylated tau protein.

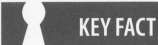

## KEY FACT

Mild Cognitive Impairment is a clinical syndrome and has a broad differential diagnosis. If Alzheimer's disease is identified as the cause (using amyloid positron emission tomography [PET] scan or cerebrospinal fluid [CSF] studies), then it is called MCI due to AD or simply "Prodromal AD."

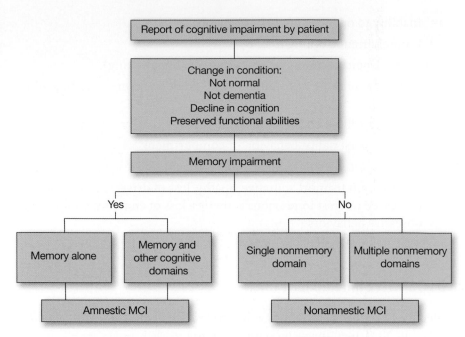

**FIGURE 6-1. Diagnostic decision tree for mild cognitive impairment.** Reproduced with permission from Rafii M. *First Aid for the Neurology Boards, 2nd ed.* New York: McGraw Hill; 2015.

- Sparse diffuse extracellular neocortical beta-amyloid plaques.
- If there is no underlying AD pathology, then other etiologies include depression, sleep apnea, medication effects, and other neurodegenerative disorders (Fig. 6-1).

**Treatment:**

- No FDA-approved treatments for MCI.
- Clinicians commonly advise their patients to maintain a healthy diet and engage in new or even old hobbies/activities that require learning and facilitate critical thinking.

## ALZHEIMER'S DISEASE (AD)

**Late onset vs early onset:**

- Late Onset is the AD we typically think of when we discuss AD.
- Early Onset (begins before age 65) is different from late-onset AD, especially in its degree of genetic predisposition and different, often nonamnestic, phenotypic presentation.

**Epidemiology:**

- Most common dementia in the United States.
- Prevalence is about 5.7 million in the United States; 80% are >75 years old.
- Incidence increases with age: 2 per 1000 at ages 65 to 74, 37/1000 at 85 or older.
- Number of patients with AD in the United States projected to nearly triple by 2050 with majority of growth attributed to those >85 years old.
- Two-thirds of AD patients are women, reflecting increased life duration in addition to biological factors.
- Compared to non-Hispanic White people, incidence is higher in African American/Black and Hispanic/Latinx people and lower in Asian American people.

- Progression in three stages: (1) Preclinical, (2) MCI due to AD, and (3) Dementia due to AD.
- Survival rate (from day of diagnosis):
  - Four to eight years in those diagnosed at an older age, with psychotic features, motor system involvement, or medical comorbidities.
  - Up to 15 to 20 years in the otherwise healthy.

**Risk factors:**

- Age (strongest factor for regular AD).
- Family history of dementia (strongest factor for early onset AD).
- Environmental:
  - Vascular injury (eg, stroke).
  - Sleep disturbances (insomnia, obstructive sleep apnea, poor sleep quality, working night shifts).
  - Traumatic brain injury (TBI).
  - Late life depression:
    - Unclear if risk factor or consequence of AD in serotonergic and noradrenergic brainstem nuclei.
  - Fewer years of formal education.
  - Lack of moderate- to high-intensity exercise.
  - Lack of social engagement.
- Genetic:
  - Late-onset AD has heritability of 60% to 80% with strongest genetic risk factor being the APOE gene.
    - Apolipoprotein E (APOE)—encodes the brain's major cholesterol transporter and has three major alleles: e2, e3, e4.
      - APOE e4 contributes most to development of AD with e4/e4 homozygosity having the greatest predisposition.
      - APOE e2 is protective.
    - >20 additional genes, including TREM2 (triggering receptor expressed on myeloid cells 2).
    - Autosomal Dominant AD: Mutations in presenilin 1 (PSEN1) on chr. 14, presenilin 2 (PSEN2) on chr. 1, and amyloid prescursor protein (APP) on chr. 21 lead to early onset dementia.
    - All persons with Down syndrome (Trisomy 21) have an extra copy of APP gene and therefore have a high risk for AD dementia by age 55.

**Approaching patients with suspected AD:**

- Obtain corroborative information from family members, close friends, PCPs, etc., since patient recall will be limited.
- Focused history looking for deficits in the following domains:
  - Early and prominent deficits in episodic memory.
    - Difficulty recalling recent events and sparing of remote memory.
    - On memory tests, patients show impaired learning, rapid forgetting, and poor delayed recall (dysfunction of hippocampal circuit).
  - Executive, language, and visuospatial impairment.
  - Changes in motor, autonomic, sleep, dietary, and emotional function and social behavior.
  - Review medical comorbidities, medications, substance use, and environmental exposures.

**KEY FACT**

**Age is the biggest risk factor for Alzheimer's disease.**

- Montreal Cognitive Assessment (MOCA) or Mini Mental Status Exam (MMSE).
- Labs to rule out reversible causes of changes in cognition:
  - CBC, electrolytes (specifically, Na), LFTs, Ammonia level, renal function (uremia), thyroid function tests, B12, folate, RPR.
- CT or MRI brain without contrast to exclude structural lesions and examine vascular injury.
  - MRI can also be helpful in identifying characteristic patterns of *brain atrophy* and white matter injury (Fig. 6-2).

## Pathophysiology:

- Senile plaques: extracellular deposits of aggregated amyloid-B polypeptides.
  - First in neocortex, then spread successively into hippocampus and limbic structures, striatum and diencephalon, brainstem, and cerebellum.
- Neurofibrillary tangles: aggregated, hyperphosphorylated forms of the microtubule binding protein tau.
  - Distribution of tangles: first in entorhinal cortex, followed by limbic, then cortical regions.
- Cognitive symptoms correlate more with burden of neurofibrillary tangles than with amyloid plaques.
- In older patients with AD, Lewy body pathology, TDP-43 inclusions, and hippocampal sclerosis pathologies are commonly found in tandem with AD pathology, especially >90 years old.
- AD associated with *loss of cholinergic neurons in basal forebrain*, the primary target for pharmacological treatment of AD.

## Evaluation:

- MRI:
  - Atrophy of hippocampus and medial temporal lobes (seen best on T1).
  - Temporoparietal cortical atrophy.
  - Ventricular enlargement.
  - Greater medial temporal atrophy and less cortical atrophy than in early-onset AD.
  - T2 FLAIR hyperintensities which are nonspecific but associated with small vessel ischemic disease.

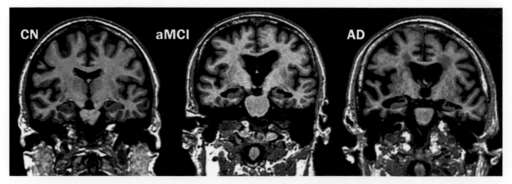

**FIGURE 6-2. Progressive atrophy (medial temporal lobes) in an older cognitively normal (CN) subject, an amnestic mild cognitive impairment (aMCI) subject, and an Alzheimer's disease (AD) subject.** Reproduced with permission from Vemuri, P., Jack, C.R. Role of structural MRI in Alzheimer's disease. Alz Res Therapy 2, 23 (2010).

- On some sequences may show cortical microbleeds ("superficial siderosis") suggestive of cerebral amyloid angiopathy (CAA) which can co-occur with AD.
- Functional brain imaging with fludeoxyglucose positron emission tomography (FDG-PET):
  - Reduced metabolism on FDG-PET in temporoparietal cortex and posterior cingulate/precuneus.
  - Amyloid and Tau PET imaging are still more widely used in the research realm.
- Lumbar puncture:
  - Amyloid-beta low in CSF implies elevated brain amyloid.
  - Total Tau (t-tau) and phosphorylated tau (p-tau) are elevated in CSF and still in the research realm.

**Treatment:**

- AD-specific medications, treatment of vascular risk factors, sleep disorders, mood disorders, comorbid conditions, counseling about safety and future planning, and referrals to community resources.
- Acetylcholinesterase inhibitors (AChEI):
  - Symptomatic benefit in cognitive and functional outcomes for mild-to-severe AD (no benefit in MCI)—manifests as slower/less decline.
  - Also help with depression, anxiety, apathy, and abhorrent motor behaviors:
    - Donepezil.
    - Galantine.
    - Rivastigmine.
    - Adverse effects: GI upset, loss of appetite, urinary frequency, muscle cramps, vivid dreams, slowing of cardiac conduction (caution in patients with bradycardia).
- NMDA-R antagonists:
  - Memantine is used for moderate-to-severe AD.
  - Improve agitation, lability, and irritability.
  - Adverse effects: Constipation, dizziness, HA, somnolence.
  - Use AChEI in mild AD and *add* Memantine in moderate AD.
- SSRI/SNRI:
  - Depression and agitation.
- Melatonin for sleep.
- Medications to avoid:
  - Tricyclic antidepressants (TCAs) due to their anticholinergic effects.
  - Typical AND atypical antipsychotics.
  - Benzodiazepines as they are sedating and can worsen cognition. Can cause agitation in elderly as well.
- Anti-amyloid monoclonal antibodies.
  - Mechanism—Remove amyloid plaques. Given IV. Risk of cerebral edema or microhemorrhages.
- Aducanumab.
- Lecanemab.

### TABLE 6-1. Symptoms Associated with Neurodegenerative Dementia

| Episodic Memory | Psychiatric/Behavioral |
|---|---|
| • Forgetting recent events<br>• Misplacing personal items<br>• Asking repetitive questions<br>• Missing appointments<br>• Paying the bills late<br>• Poor long-term/autobiographical memory | • Depression<br>• Apathy<br>• Anxiety<br>• Irritability<br>• Agitation<br>• Poor impulse control, lability<br>• Delusions<br>• Hallucinations or misperceptions<br>• Changes in personality<br>• New hobbies or interests<br>• Obsessive or compulsive behaviors<br>• Loss of empathy<br>• Disinhibition<br>• Poor hygiene |
| Visuospatial | Language |
| • Navigational problems/getting lost<br>• Difficulty locating items in plain sight<br>• Problems visually recognizing faces or objects | • Difficulty retrieving words or names<br>• Problems comprehending words or sentences<br>• Effortful or nonfluent speech<br>• Grammar errors or omissions<br>• Spelling errors<br>• Problems reading and writing |
| Executive Function | Motor |
| • Problems organizing, multitasking, or maintaining focus<br>• Distractibility<br>• Difficulty reasoning, problem solving, or making decisions<br>• Poor judgment | • Repetitive/restless behavior<br>• Muscle weakness<br>• Poor balance/falls<br>• Problems using hands or feet<br>• Incoordination<br>• Tremor or other adventitial movements<br>• Muscle cramps<br>• Fasciculations |
| Sleep | General and Autonomic |
| • Insomnia<br>• Loud snoring/gasping for air<br>• Dream enactment behavior | • Weight loss or gain<br>• Changes in eating behavior and dietary preferences<br>• Positional dizziness<br>• Bladder or bowel incontinence<br>• Sexual dysfunction |
| Other | |
| • Problems with calculations<br>• Difficulty using devise/technology<br>• Disorientation to time and place | |

## LEWY BODY DISEASE (LBD)

Lewy Body Disease is an umbrella term that includes Parkinson Disease (PD) Dementia and Dementia with Lewy Bodies (DLB). It is the second most common degenerative dementia after AD.

- PD Dementia: Dementia occurring in the context of an established diagnosis of PD.

- Dementia with Lewy Bodies: Dementia associated with some combination of fluctuating cognition, recurrent visual hallucinations, rapid eye movement (REM) sleep behavior disorder (RBD), and parkinsonism starting with or after the dementia diagnosis.

■ Lewy Body Disease: A pathologic diagnosis based purely on the identification of Lewy body pathology on postmortem examination independent of clinical presentation.

• **Lewy bodies** = **alpha-synuclein** inclusions.

## DLB diagnosis:

■ Dementia with early and prominent deficits in attention, executive function, and visuoperceptual ability; prominent/persistent memory impairment occurs with progression.

■ Recurrent visual hallucinations.

■ *REM sleep behavior disorder* (may precede other symptoms):

• 75% of people with RBD are diagnosed with a synuclein-related neurode-generative disease after 10 years (Table 6-1).

■ Parkinsonism—defined as one or more spontaneous cardinal features: *bradykinesia, postural instability rest tremor, rigidity.*

• Supportive features: insensitivity to antipsychotic agents, postural instability, repeated falls, syncope or other transient episodes of unresponsiveness, severe autonomic dysfunction (constipation, orthostatic hypotension, urinary incontinence).

• Hypersomnia/excessive daytime sleepiness or hyposomnia.

• Nonvisual hallucinations.

• Systematized delusions.

• Apathy, anxiety, and depression.

## PD dementia diagnosis:

■ Prevalence of dementia in PD is 25% to 30%, typically years after motor symptoms emerge.

■ Male predominance.

■ Mostly sporadic:

• ~10% inherited in autosomal-dominant pattern (**alpha-synuclein mutation).**

• Rarely autosomal-recessive pattern with mutations in *parkin* gene.

• DJ-1 gene mutation in juvenile parkinsonism.

■ Motor symptoms: bradykinesia, rigidity, resting tremor, shuffling gait, and abnormal postural reflexes.

■ PD dementia is a "subcortical" type, characterized by slowness of mental processing, forgetfulness, impaired cognition, apathy, and depression.

• These patients have less severe intellectual and memory dysfunction and lack the aphasia, agnosia, and apraxia seen in typical cortical dementias.

• Also seen are anxiety and visual hallucinations (the latter of which can be worsened by supplemental dopamine).

■ Cognitive symptoms: most patients experience cognitive impairment (dementia or MCI) after 15 to 20 years.

■ Criteria for diagnosis:

• Parkinson disease diagnosis.

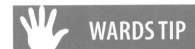

**WARDS TIP**

In DLB, hallucinations, dementia, and parkinsonism occur at around the same time, whereas in PD dementia, motor symptoms present first, and hallucinations and dementia after about 2 years.

- Dementia with impairment in more than one cognitive domain.
    - Impaired attention, executive function, bradyphrenia, visuospatial function.
    - Impaired memory: free recall of recent events and learning new material, usually improving with cueing; recognition typically better than free recall.
    - Language is usually preserved, but word-finding difficulties and impaired complex sentence comprehension may be present.
- Behavioral features:
    - Apathy.
    - Depression, anxiety.
    - Hallucinations (usually visual and consisting of complex, formed visions of people, animals, or objects).
    - Delusions (usually paranoid).
    - Excessive daytime sleepiness.

Historically, presence of dementia within the first year of onset of parkinsonian symptoms suggested a diagnosis of DLB instead of PD. In 2015, this rule was nulled. Now, PD is diagnosed based on criteria (see Chapter 8) and can be further categorized as having *PD, Dementia with Lewy Bodies Subtype.*

In DLB, parkinsonian symptoms develop on average 2 years after onset of dementia. Motor symptoms are milder in DLB but may respond less well to medication.

### Treatment for symptomatic LBD:

- No FDA-approved medications for DLB.
- Use of cholinesterase inhibitors in LBD and PD dementia.
    - Rivastigmine-only is approved for PD dementia.
- Discuss safety concerns (eg, driving), assessing pain, screening for and managing behavioral and psychiatric symptoms, advanced care planning, and palliative care counseling.
- Avoid benzodiazepines, anticholinergic/antimuscarinics, antipsychotics, and tricyclics.
    - Antipsychotics come with risk of hypersensitivity reactions (eg, sudden deterioration, severe parkinsonism, and mental status changes—confusion to unresponsive).
- PD Dementia:
    - Anticholinergics for tremor (trihexyphenidyl, benztropine):
        - Dopamine agonists and amantadine are associated with worsened cognition and with psychosis.
    - PD psychosis does not need to be treated if not troublesome.
        - Can be with Pimavanserin (though elderly at risk for death; also may prolong QT interval).
- Melatonin for RBD:
    - Clonazepam cautious second line.

- Orthostatic hypotension: wean contributing meds, eg, dopamine agonists, anti-HTN; midodrine, fludrocortisone, droxidopa, increased water/salt intake, compression stockings.
- Sialorrhea—botulinum toxin, glycopyrrolate, ipratropium bromide sublingual spray, atropine sublingual drops.
- Nonpharmacologic treatments:
  - Moderate- to high-intensity exercise, physical therapy, occupational therapy, and speech therapy.

## BEHAVIORAL VARIANT (BV) OF FRONTOTEMPORAL DEMENTIA (FTD)

Belongs to class of FTDs which are united by underlying *frontotemporal* lobar degeneration due to accumulation of **tau neurofibrillary tangles**.

Social and emotional functions slowly decline in BvFTD. It is the most common type of FTD and is a devastating neurodegenerative syndrome with mean age onset 58 years and range of 20 to 90+ years old.

**Symptoms:**

- Subtle changes in behavior that may be mistaken for "midlife crisis," depression, etc.
- Recurrent job loss and unanticipated marital discord are common complaints.
- Spouse's major life event (eg, cancer diagnosis) may be ignored or trivialized.
- Core features:
  - Apathy: Loss of motivation toward previously valued interests and activities.
  - **Disinhibition**.
  - Loss of sympathy, empathy, compassion, social grace.
  - Repetitive and compulsive and ritualistic behaviors.
  - Predilection for sweets and relentless overeating (hyperorality and dietary changes).
- Abandon family duties.
- Approach strangers (including children) with unwanted questions or other interpersonal boundary violations.
- Tactlessly comment on others' weight, attractiveness, etc.

Earliest and most consistent atrophy is of the anterior cingulate cortex, anterior insula, striatum, amygdala, hypothalamus, and thalamus. These make up the salience network which processes internal and external stimuli to elicit the proper visceral-emotional-autonomic, behavioral, and cognitive responses (Table 6-2).

The following changes in behavior are linked to specific brain regions:
- Dorsolateral prefrontal cortex: executive dysfunction, distractibility, disorganization, mental rigidity
- Right > left anterior temporal lobe: semantic loss, especially emotions and faces
- Left anterior midcingulate and presupplementary motor area: Abulia, adynamic aphasia
- Entorhinal-hippocampal complex: memory loss

**KEY FACT**

Must be distinguished from Alzheimer-type dementia in which frontal/neuropsychiatric features do arise.

**TABLE 6-2. Other Causes of Dementia**

| | |
|---|---|
| Vitamin deficiencies<br>    Thiamine B1 (Wernicke encephalopathy)<br>    B12 (eg, pernicious anemia)<br>    Nicotinic acid (pellagra) | Toxic<br>    Drug, medication, narcotic poisoning<br>    Heavy metal intoxication<br>    Dialysis dementia—thought to be re-<br>        versible after kidney transplant<br>    Organic toxins |
| Endocrine and other organ failure<br>    Hypothyroidism<br>    Adrenal insufficiency<br>    Cushing syndrome<br>    Renal failure<br>    Liver failure<br>    Pulmonary failure | Chronic infections<br>    HIV<br>    Neurosyphilis<br>    Prion disease<br>    Tuberculosis, fungal, protozoal<br>    Sarcoidosis<br>    Whipple Disease |
| Degenerative<br>    Huntington Disease<br>    Progressive supranuclear palsy<br>    Corticobasal degeneration<br>    Multiple systems atrophy<br>    Hereditary Ataxias<br>    Motor neuron disease (eg, ALS)<br>    Multiple Sclerosis | Head trauma and diffuse brain damage<br>    Dementia pugilistica<br>    Chronic subdural hemorrhage<br>    Post-anoxia<br>    Postencephalitic<br>    Normal pressure hydrocephalus |
| Neoplastic<br>    Primary and metastatic brain tumors<br>    Paraneoplastic limbic encephalitis | Other<br>    Vasculitis<br>    CADASIL<br>    Acute intermittent porphyria<br>    Recurrent nonconvulsive seizures<br>    Transient epileptic amnesia<br>    Obstructive Sleep Apnea |
| Psychiatric<br>    Depression<br>    Schizophrenia<br>    Conversion reaction | Medications<br>    Narcotics<br>    Benzodiazepines<br>    Anticholinergics |

- Substantia nigra, striatum: motor impairment that may include parkinsonism
- Frontal eye fields, dorsal midbrain: oculomotor control problems
- UMN and LMN: motor neuron disease
- Lateral posterior parietal cortex: alexia, agraphia, acalculia, anomia, visuospatial dysfunction (mostly in inherited BvFTD)

**Genetics:**

- Major genes involved: MAPT, GRN, C90orf72
- Autosomal dominant in up to one-fifth of patients
- Three major protein deposits: tau, TDP-43, and fused sarcoma

**Diagnosis:**

- Involves a good history, like with all dementias.
- Neuropsychological testing to determine which domains are malfunctioning:
  - Link changes in behavior found on neuropsychological testing with atrophy in the associated brain regions.
  - Rule out psychiatric disease, vascular disease (frontal strokes), substance abuse, frontotemporal brain sagging syndrome from prolonged hypotension.

- MRI findings:
  - Anterior-predominant pattern of atrophy, usually including the anterior insula and anterior cingulate cortices.
- FDG PET less metabolism in frontal and anterior temporal regions.

**Treatment:**

- No disease modifying therapies available.
- Caregiver support, behavioral management.
- Symptomatic behavioral control:
  - SSRI: overeating, compulsivity.
  - Venlafaxine: for apathy.
  - Atypical antipsychotics: psychosis and acute agitation causing harm to others. Caution for cardiac death.
  - Anticholinergics may worsen agitation.

## NORMAL PRESSURE HYDROCEPHALUS (NPH)

- A **triad** of dementia, gait apraxia (magnetic gait and postural instability), and urinary urgency followed by incontinence (wacky, wobbly, and wet):
  - Impaired attention and concentration measured by digit span, arithmetic, block design, and symbol/digit matching.
  - Psychomotor slowing.
  - Apathy.
  - Gait: small steps, wide based, difficulty with turns, and postural instability with positive pull test.
- A large-volume (30-50 mL of CSF) lumbar puncture is therapeutic and diagnosis is confirmed with improvement in gait 2 hours to 2 days later, but usually within 30 minutes.
  - Once diagnosis is confirmed, patient is candidate for a ventriculoperitoneal shun.
- Pathophysiology:
  - Ventricular enlargement with normal intracranial pressure:
    - Etiology is multifactorial: impaired CSF absorption, congenital causes, vascular disease.
    - <50% biopsies show arachnoid fibrosis and most show normal brain parenchyma.
  - Coexisting white matter hyperintensities/vascular disease which is consistent with prevalence of disease in elderly population.
- Evaluate for factors that may aggravate hydrocephalus: hypertension, recent head injury, sleep apnea, congestive heart failure, obesity.
- Evaluate for other causes of gait disturbance: arthritis, cervical myelopathy, visual impairment, lumbar stenosis, radiculopathy, and peripheral neuropathy.
- MRI findings:
  - **Ventriculomegaly**.
  - Relative lack of global atrophy; though global atrophy does not exclude NPH.
  - Often seen: thinning of corpus callosum, distension of third ventricle, dilated aqueduct of sylvius.

## WARDS TIP

NPH patients are "wet, wacky, and wobbly" (incontinent, confused, unsteady gait).

- CSF:
  - Metabolites of APP, t-tau, and p-tau are low and normalize after shunt is placed.
  - Elevated t-tau and p-tau can rule out NPH.

## VASCULAR COGNITIVE IMPAIRMENT

Cerebrovascular disease is a common cause of dementia and often coexists with neurodegenerative causes of dementia.

No typical presentation, as a patient can have an ischemic insult anywhere in the brain due to a myriad of reasons. For example, repeated ischemic insults to frontal lobe can present as behavioral variant frontotemporal dementia, a devastating type of dementia that must be carefully diagnosed. And those with vascular disease and AD may present as pure AD.

However, those with vascular dementia often present with executive and cognitive speed dysfunction more often than with memory issues. White matter ischemia also leads to depression and gait impairment. The decline is stepwise decline and involves focal deficits (eg, hemiparesis) from large territory strokes. Vascular dementia has an insidious onset of cognitive slowing from cerebral small vessel disease.

**Poststroke dementia** (both cortical and subcortical):
- 10% have dementia prior to their first stroke.
- 10% develop dementia shortly after first stroke.
- 33% develop dementia after a recurrent stroke.
- 28% develop dementia after lobar intracerebral hemorrhage.

**Types:**
- Multi-infarct dementia
- Small vessel dementia
- Strategic infarct dementia (targeted [by chance] infarcts to specific areas which result in profound cognitive deficits)
- Hypoperfusion dementia (cardiac arrest/anoxic injury, watershed infarcts)
- Hemorrhagic dementia
- Hereditary vascular dementia—cerebral autosomal-dominant arteriopathy with subcortical infarcts and leukoencephalopathy (CADASIL) w/ ischemia of anterior temporal lobe
- Mixed dementia—vascular and other neurodegenerative processes

**Etiologies:**
- Hypertensive arteriopathy:
  - Subcortical predilection as these small vessels are more susceptible to changes in pressure—lacunar strokes
- Cerebral amyloid angiopathy (CAA):
  - Cortical predilection as amyloid is preferentially deposited in cortical vessels
- Large vessel/thromboembolic disease:
  - Often seen in patients with metabolic syndrome or hypercoagulability

- Stroke risk factors: smoking, diabetes mellitus, hypertension, hyperlipidemia, atrial fibrillation, ESRD platelet dysfunction, and hypercoagulability secondary to an inherited cause (cancer, etc.)

**Diagnosis:**

- Hyperacute ischemic infarct, microbleeds, or hemorrhage.
- Perivascular white matter hyperintensities on T2 FLAIR represent chronic ischemic damage due to common stroke risk factors and are associated, based on size, with increased risk of stroke, dementia, worsened cognitive speed, executive function, depression, and gait impairment.
- Bilateral thalamic strokes lead to "goofy" behavior.
- CAA, even without hemorrhage, is associated with impaired episodic memory and decreased perceptual speed even in absence of coexisting AD pathology.
- Convexity subarachnoid hemorrhage: recurrent transient spreading sensory and motor symptoms.

**Treatment:**

- Symptomatic as with all dementias
- Anticholinergics and memantine for dual vascular and AD pathology
- SSRIs for depression and pseudobulbar affect
- Dextromethorphan-quinidine for pseudobulbar affect:
  - Also used in Multiple Sclerosis (MS) and amyotrophic lateral sclerosis (ALS)

**Prevention:**

- Aggressive blood pressure management
- Mediterranean diet over low-fat diet
- Lifestyle modification

# CHRONIC TRAUMATIC ENCEPHALOPATHY (CTE)

CTE is a long-term consequence of concussive and subconcussive repetitive head impact (not to be confused with Post-Concussive Syndrome). Concussions are blows/injuries to head which result in temporary memory or orientation deficits, and Post-Concussive Syndrome is constellation of signs that may remain for weeks to years and include insomnia, vertigo, tinnitus, anxiety, fatigue, and depression.

**Diagnosis:**

- The diagnosis is clinical.
  - Tau PET imaging is still on the horizon.
  - Elevated t-tau in serum is nonspecific for CTE.
  - CSF studies have not yet been shown to be diagnostic.
- History of contact sports or repetitive head trauma. Only diagnosable on autopsy.
  - Unknown mechanism but thought to be result of repeated head trauma.
  - Most symptoms occur years to decades after initial head trauma.
- Perivascular accumulations of phosphorylated tau (p-tau) in neurons and astrocytes in an irregular pattern at depths of the cortical sulci.

**Symptoms** involve cognition, behavior, and mood, though no distinct clinical criteria exist yet.

■ Impaired memory, attention executive function, concentration, judgment, problem solving.

■ Cognitive and behavioral deficits may lead to substance abuse, bankruptcy, failed relationships, and even anger/domestic abuse.

■ Sadness/depression, hopelessness, suicidal ideation/attempts.

■ Explosivity, feeling "out of control."

■ Language impairment and visuospatial difficulties.

■ Physical or verbal violence.

■ Impulse control problems.

■ Motor symptoms.

**Treatment** is symptomatic.

## PRION DISEASE

■ Prion isoform leads to misfolding within neurons and other proteins, leading to a rapidly progressive dementia.

- **Spongiform vacuolation**.
- Associated with dementia, ataxia, myoclonus, and rapid death.

■ Creutzfeldt-Jakob disease (CJD)—rapidly progressive dementia and myoclonic jerks.

- Sporadic—85% of cases. 1/1,000,000 incidence usually older than 65 years.
- Familial—autosomal dominant.
- Acquired—iatrogenic transmission (eg, brain surgery, transplantation), dietary ingestion (Mad cow disease).

■ Kuru—Associated with cannibalism endemic to Papua New Guinea.

■ Gerstmann-Sträussler-Scheinker syndrome—Inherited, primarily affects cerebellum. Causes dysarthria, truncal ataxia, and progressive dementia.

**MRI findings:**

■ **"Hockey-stick"** sign—T2 FLAIR hyperintensity of dorsomedial and posterior thalamic nuclei.

■ Also see T2 changes in periaqueductal gray matter and head of the caudate (Fig. 6-3).

**EEG findings:**

■ Triphasic periodic sharp and slow-wave complexes (PSCWs) are characteristic of CJD.

**Lumbar puncture:**

■ 14-3-3 protein

■ RT-QuIC test in CSF

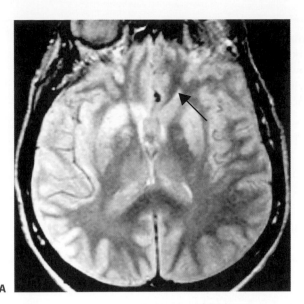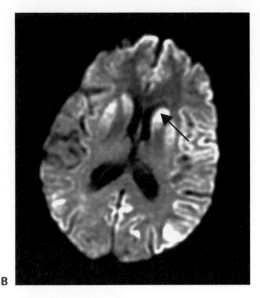

A B

**FIGURE 6-3. Typical brain MRI findings of a patient with Creutzfeldt-Jakob disease demonstrating T2 and DWI signal changes in the basal ganglia and cortical ribbon.**
Reproduced, with permission, from Ropper AH, Brown RH. *Adams and Victor's Principles of Neurology*, 8th ed. New York: McGraw-Hill; 2005: 655.

 **Case 1:** An 88-year-old male with history of hypertension and diabetes is brought in by family for new-onset confusion. The patient is mumbling and wanting to go home but is not oriented to place or time. No focal weakness or sensory deficits are found on exam. A bedside sitter was assigned to ensure frequent reorientation and prevent unsafe ambulation as he is at risk of tripping over his lines and falling. The patient's vitals are unremarkable, while the urinalysis reveals increased leukocyte and nitrite levels as well as an increased white count and bacteria.

What is the diagnosis?

A. Delirium secondary to a UTI
B. Progression of dementia
C. Stroke
D. Failure to thrive

The correct answer is A. Delirium secondary to a UTI.

 **Case 2:** A 79-year-old woman has a 2-year history of memory loss and occasional confusion along with a slow and unsteady gait. There is no evidence of focal weakness or rigidity. She has also developed urinary incontinence. MRI shows enlarged ventricles but no significant cerebral atrophy. The best treatment is which of the following?

A. Cholinesterase inhibitor
B. Physical therapy
C. L-dopa
D. Ventricular-peritoneal shunt

The correct answer is D. She has normal pressure hydrocephalus based on exam and MRI. A large volume LP would help confirm the diagnosis and a VP shunt would be the most appropriate treatment.

**Case 3:** A 58-year-old male has a 6-month history of confusion, forgetfulness, and myoclonic jerks. His family denies any travel, recent surgery, or other illnesses. CSF shows 14-3-3 protein and MRI shows cortical ribbon of restricted diffusion. His history is notable for receiving injections of cadaveric growth hormone for short stature as a child. What is the most likely diagnosis?

A. Acquired CJD
B. Schizophrenia
C. Behavioral-variant frontotemporal dementia (BvFTD)
D. Lewy body dementia

The correct answer is A. The cadaveric growth hormone was likely from a patient with sporadic CJD and led to transmission of the prion protein via injection.

# CHAPTER 7

# MULTIPLE SCLEROSIS AND DEMYELINATING DISEASES

In this chapter, we will cover multiple sclerosis (MS) and other demyelinating diseases. With recent advances, MS can be much more easily diagnosed and managed as a chronic disease. It will be important to know about MS variants and their differences.

## Multiple Sclerosis

### DEFINITION AND EPIDEMIOLOGY

- MS affects about 1 in every 750 people in the United States, which means there are currently about 400,000 Americans living with the illness.
  - Around the world, there are about 2.5 million people with the disease. More recent research suggests that these numbers are a vast underestimate, and that nearly 1 million people have MS in the United States alone.
- MS typically affects people between the ages of 15 and 40, although occasionally, people are diagnosed outside of this age range.
  - Predominantly affects women, with a 2.5:1 ratio to men.
- Can occur in different forms but 85% of cases are relapsing-remitting form (Fig. 7-1 and Table 7-1).

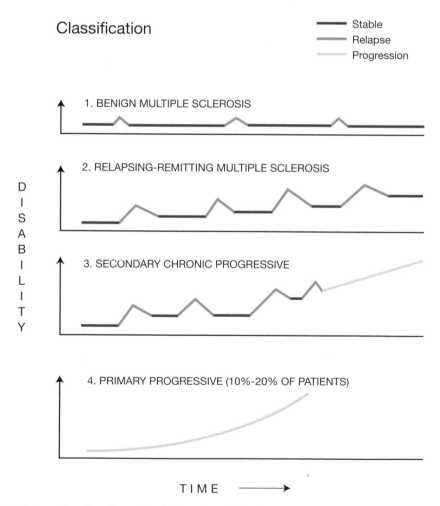

**FIGURE 7-1. Classification of multiple sclerosis by disease course.** Reproduced with permission from Rafii MS., Cochrane TI. *First Aid for the Neurology Boards. 2nd ed.* New York: McGraw Hill; 2015.

**TABLE 7-1. McDonald Criteria for MS Diagnosis (2010)**

| Clinical (Attack) | Lesions | Additional Criteria to Make Diagnosis |
|---|---|---|
| 2 or more | Objective clinical evidence of 2 or more lesions or objective clinical evidence of 1 lesion with reasonable historical evidence of a prior attack | None. Clinical evidence alone will suffice; additional evidence desirable but must be consistent with MS |
| 2 or more | Objective clinical evidence of 1 lesion | Dissemination in space, demonstrated by<br>• 1 T2 lesion in at least 2 MS typical CNS regions (periventricular, juxtacortical, infratentorial, spinal cord); OR<br>• Await further clinical attack implicating a different CNS site |
| 1 | Objective clinical evidence of 2 or more lesions | Dissemination in time, demonstrated by simultaneous asymptomatic contrast-enhancing and nonenhancing lesions at any time; OR<br>• A new T2 and/or contrast-enhancing lesion(s) on follow-up MRI, irrespective of its timing; OR<br>• Await a second clinical attack |
| 1 | Objective clinical evidence of 1 lesion | Dissemination in space, demonstrated by<br>• 1 T2 lesion in at least 2 MS typical CNS regions (periventricular, juxtacortical, infratentorial, spinal cord); OR<br>• Await further clinical attack implicating a different CNS site AND dissemination in time, demonstrated by<br>• Simultaneous asymptomatic contrast-enhancing and non-enhancing lesions at any time; OR<br>• A new T2 and/or contrast-enhancing lesion(s) on follow-up MRI, irrespective of its timing; OR<br>• Await a second clinical attack |
| 0 | Progression from the onset | One year of disease progression (retrospective or prospective) AND at least 2 out of 3 criteria:<br>• Dissemination in space in the brain based on 1 T2 lesion in periventricular, juxtacortical, or infratentorial regions;<br>• Dissemination in space in the spinal cord based on 2 T2 lesions; OR<br>• Positive CSF |

Reproduced with permission from Polman CH, Reingold SC, Banwell B, et al. *Diagnostic criteria for multiple sclerosis: 2010 revisions to the McDonald Criteria. Ann Neurol.* 2011;69(2):292–302.

## ETIOLOGY

- Multifactorial with a slight genetic component
- Various immunogenic triggers implicated
  - Viruses (EBV, HSV)
  - Bacteria (*Chlamydia pneumoniae*, mycoplasma)
  - Prevalence decreases with proximity to equator at birth

## SIGNS AND SYMPTOMS

- **Optic neuritis**: usually unilateral, painful, and an early manifestation.
- Spinal cord demyelination: spasticity, hyperreflexia, positive Babinski, impaired gait, loss of sensation, weakness, numbness.
- Cerebellar involvement: poor postural control, tremor, lack of coordination.
- Cranial nerve palsies: diplopia, facial palsy.
- Autonomic dysfunction: bladder, bowel, and sexual dysfunction.
- **Medial Longitudinal Fasciculus syndrome:** internuclear ophthalmoplegia (impaired adduction of ipsilateral eye; nystagmus of contralateral eye with abduction).

**WARDS TIP**

Uhthoff phenomenon triggered by fever associated with viral illness may be confused with MS exacerbation.

- **Lhermitte sign:** cervical spine damage with electrical pain or tingling when the neck is flexed. Pain radiates from neck down the spine. Pain may also radiate into arms or legs.
- **Uhthoff phenomenon:** when a patient with demyelinating disease (eg, multiple sclerosis) experiences recrudescence of symptoms from an existing CNS lesion due to an increase in body temperature. Increase in body temperature may be from fever, exercise, or high ambient temperatures (eg, hot bath).

## DIAGNOSIS

Dissemination in time and space. This means one clinical episode with objective evidence of neurologic disease (demonstrated via either MRI or CSF) plus evidence of a second episode demonstrated again either by magnetic resonance imaging (MRI) criteria, positive spinal fluid findings, or abnormal evoked potentials.

- **CSF:**
  - Presence of oligoclonal IgG bands
  - Elevated IgG index
  - Lymphocyte pleocytosis <50/mm³
  - Increased immunoglobulin G (IgG) synthesis
  - Increased myelin basic protein (MBP)
- **MRI:**
  - Gadolinium (Gd)-enhanced scans:
    - Multiple sclerotic plaques seen in periventricular white matter areas.
    - Demonstration of blood-brain barrier breakdown.
    - Indicative of acute inflammatory activity within CNS.
    - Usually resolves within 4 to 6 weeks.
  - T1-hypointense scans ("black holes"):
    - Indicate serious brain injury.
    - Reflect chronic MS lesions with localized areas of axonal loss and gliosis.
    - Provide better correlation of disability in SPMS than T2-hyperintense lesions.
    - A subset of T2-hyperintense lesions become black holes (Fig. 7-2).

## TREATMENT

- Acute attacks (eg, optic neuritis) treated with IV methylprednisolone or plasmapharesis
- Disease-modifying treatments:
  - Dimethyl fumarate - Oral immunosuppressant
  - Fingolimod - Oral immunosuppressant
  - Ocrelizumab- IV anti-CD20 monoclonal antibody, immunosuppressant
  - Alemtuzumab - IV anti-CD52 monoclonal antibody, immunosuppressant
- IFNs used in MS: Recombinant proteins IFN-β1b (Betaseron) and 2 formulations of IFN-β1a (Avonex and Rebif).
- Do not cross the blood-brain barrier (BBB)—effects occur in the periphery (eg, lymphoid organs).

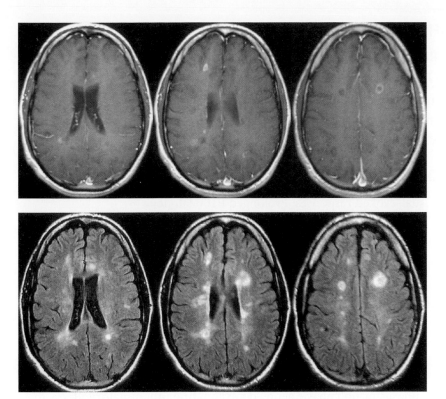

**FIGURE 7-2. Black holes seen on MRI indicating areas of previous demyelination.** Contrast-enhanced T1-weighted images show several areas of contrast uptake in acute multiple sclerosis plaques and areas of T1 hypointensity (black holes). Reproduced with permission from John C.M. Brust, *CURRENT Diagnosis & Treatment: Neurology, 3e.* New York: Copyright © 2019 by McGraw-Hill Education. All rights reserved. Figure 17.3.

- *Glatiramer acetate* (Copaxone) is a polypeptide mixture with peripheral and CNS effects. It may work by blocking autoimmune T cells, inducing anergy, anti-inflammatory Th2 cells, and bystander suppression.

- Natalizumab: Monoclonal antibody against α4-integrin that inhibits leukocyte adhesion and migration into brain and spinal cord.

  - Risk of multifocal leukoencephalopathy:

    - Test for antibodies to JC virus before initiating therapy.

## Optic Neuritis

Acute or subacute inflammation of the optic nerve with visual loss. Often associated with or presenting symptoms of multiple sclerosis.

### SYMPTOMS

- Loss of vision (mostly central vision) is affected.
- Color vision is impaired.
- Orbital pain with eye movement is common.

### EXAM

- Reduced visual acuity of the affected eye
- Relative afferent papillary defect (RAPD)—ipsilateral pupil
- Brisk consensual response to light in the unaffected eye, but poor response to direct light
- Inflamed optic nerve head
- Red color desaturation

## DIFFERENTIAL DIAGNOSIS

- Retinal or macular disease
- Granulomatous (sarcoidosis)
- Tumors (lymphoma, glioma, melanoma, metastatic foci)
- Infectious (fungal)
- Vasculitis

## ADDITIONAL TESTS

- Visual-evoked responses: Prolonged P100 latency
- Visual field defect
- Color vision defect
- Post-gadolinium T1 enhancement in optic nerve

## TREATMENT

- Intravenous methylprednisolone 1 g/d × 3-5 days

## Acute Disseminated Encephalomyelitis (ADEM)

Monophasic, or polyphasic acute, demyelinating inflammatory illness that typically follows upper respiratory infection (50%-75%) or vaccination. More common in children. Symptoms first appear 7 to 14 days post infection, and most are hospitalized within a week.

## SIGNS AND SYMPTOMS

- Children > adults: Prolonged fever, headache, imbalance/gait instability, dysphagia/dysarthria, diplopia
- Adults > children: Limb paresthesia and weakness

## GENERAL CLINICAL FEATURES

- First clinical attack of inflammatory or demyelinating disease in the CNS.
- Acute or subacute onset.
- Affects multifocal areas of the CNS.
- Encephalopathy: Acute behavioral change such as confusion or irritability and/or alteration in consciousness ranging from somnolence or coma.
- Attack is usually be followed by improvement in clinical and/or neuroradiologic (MRI) findings.
- Sequelae may include residual deficits.
- No other etiologies can explain the event.
- ADEM relapses (with new or fluctuating symptoms, signs, or MRI findings) occurring within 3 months of the inciting ADEM episode are considered part of the same acute event. In addition, ADEM relapses that occur during a steroid taper or within 4 weeks of completing a steroid taper are considered part of the initial inciting ADEM episode.
- **Lesion characteristics on MRI FLAIR and T2-weighted images:**
  - Large (>1-2 cm in size) multifocal, hyperintense, bilateral, asymmetric lesions in the supratentorial or infratentorial white matter. Rarely, brain MRI shows a single, large (≥1-2 cm) lesion predominantly affecting white matter.

- Gray matter, especially basal ganglia and thalamus, may be involved.
- Spinal cord MRI may show confluent intramedullary lesion(s) with variable enhancement, in addition to the abnormalities on brain MRI.
- No radiologic evidence of previous destructive white matter changes.

## DIFFERENTIAL DIAGNOSIS

- Viral, bacterial, or parasitic meningoencephalitis (Herpes simplex encephalitis is a frequent clinical mimic.)
- Other vasculitic/autoimmune conditions:
  - Initial presentation of antiphospholipid antibody syndrome
  - Primary CNS angiitis
  - Systemic lupus erythematosus (SLE)-related vasculitis
  - Neurosarcoidosis
  - Behçet disease
  - Primary or metastatic CNS neoplastic disease

## TREATMENT

- IV corticosteroids
- Oral immunosuppressants
- Plasmapheresis
- IVIG
- Cytotoxic chemotherapy

## PROGNOSIS

- Full recovery in >70%.
- Ten to 20% mild-moderate disability.
- Five percent mortality.
- Sudden severe polysymptomatic onset implies worse prognosis.

**Case 1:** A 55-year-old insurance broker receives the influenza vaccine. A few weeks later, he notices right arm weakness and slurred speech. A few days after this, he develops confusion and within 1 week, he is intubated and in a coma. MRI of the brain shows diffuse cerebral demyelination. He is started on steroids and about 6 weeks later, he begins to recover from the coma and within 3 months is fully recovered. What is the diagnosis?

A. Cortical-basilar degeneration
B. Acute disseminated encephalomyelitis (ADEM)
C. Multiple sclerosis
D. Progressive supranuclear palsy (PSP)
E. Status epilepticus

The correct answer is B. This patient had acute disseminated encephalomyelitis. This is a demyelinating disease of the brain, brainstem, and spinal cord that is indistinguishable from MS on MRI. However, it is monophasic and not relapsing and remitting like MS. It usually develops within days or weeks of a viral illness or an immunization.

**Case 2:** A 19-year-old woman develops painful eye movement and loss of vision in the right eye. She has no other symptoms or complaints. These symptoms last for 4 weeks and then seem to resolve spontaneously. What is the most likely diagnosis?

A. Optic neuritis
B. Amaurosis Fugax
C. Idiopathic intracranial hypertension
D. Atypical migraine
E. Glaucoma

The correct answer is A. Optic neuritis is the appropriate choice. Amaurosis is caused by transient ischemia of the retina due to carotid disease. IIH symptoms include headache and bilateral vision loss. Migraine and glaucoma do not cause painful eye movements.

**Case 3:** A 56-year-old female with MS develops acute weakness in all for extremities after taking a hot bath. She is so weak that she needs to call for assistance to get out of the tub. What is this phenomenon called?

A. Uhthoff phenomenon
B. Lhermitte sign
C. MLF syndrome
D. Chronic fatigue syndrome

The correct answer is A. Uhthoff's phenomenon. Lhermitte sign: Damage to the cervical spine: electrical pain or tingling when the neck is flexed. Pain radiates from neck down the spine. Pain may also radiate into arms or legs. **Uhthoff phenomenon:** When a patient with demyelinating disease (eg, multiple sclerosis) experiences recrudescence of symptoms from an existing CNS lesion due to an increase in body temperature. Increase in body temperature may be from fever, exercise, or high ambient temperatures (eg, hot bath). MLF syndrome also called internuclear ophthalmoplegia is eye movement abnormality due to demyelination of the medial longitudinal fasciculus.

# MOVEMENT DISORDERS

In this chapter, we will briefly review basal ganglia anatomy before moving into the various disorders that arise from its dysfunction, namely movement disorders. It is important to keep in mind that there are a number of diseases that appear similar but are in fact due to very different pathophysiology and therefore require different treatment strategies.

## Basal Ganglia Anatomy

The "basal ganglia" refers to a group of subcortical nuclei responsible primarily for motor control and other roles such as motor learning, executive functions and behaviors, and emotions. Basal ganglia are strongly interconnected with the cerebral cortex, thalamus, and brainstem, and several other brain areas including the limbic system. Disruption of the basal ganglia network forms the basis for several movement disorders. The main components of the basal ganglia—as defined functionally—are the striatum, consisting of both the dorsal (caudate and putamen) and ventral (nucleus accumbens and olfactory tubercle) striatum, globus pallidus, substantia nigra, and subthalamic nucleus.

The basal ganglia and related nuclei can be broadly categorized as follows:

1. **Input nuclei**
   a. Input nuclei are those structures receiving incoming information from different sources, mainly cortical, thalamic, and nigral in origin.
   b. The caudate nucleus (CN), putamen (Put), and accumbens nucleus (Acb) are all considered input nuclei (Fig. 8-1).
2. **Output nuclei**
   a. The output nuclei are those structures that send basal ganglia information to the thalamus and consist of the internal segment of the globus pallidus (GPi) and the substantia nigra pars reticulata (SNpr).

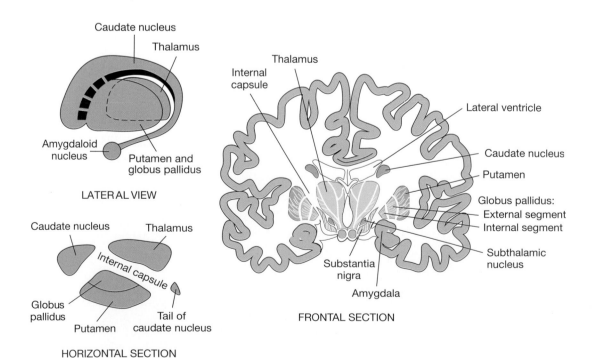

**FIGURE 8-1. Basal ganglia.** Reproduced with permission from *Ganong's Review of Medical Physiology, 26th ed.* New York: McGraw-Hill, 2019.

3. **Intrinsic nuclei**
   a. Intrinsic nuclei such as the external segment of the globus pallidus
      (GPe), the subthalamic nuclei (STN), and the substantia nigra pars
      compacta (SNpc) are located between the input and output nuclei in the
      relay of information.

## Motor Pathways

- **Direct pathway:** Projections from the caudate and putamen to the GPi and
  SNr. These are **excitatory pathways** that release the upper motor neurons
  from tonic inhibition.

  - Cortical input to the striatum stimulates it to release GABA which inhib-
    its the GPi and prevents it from releasing more GABA. Decreased GABA
    levels release the thalamus from inhibition (increases motion). This path-
    way is summarized in Fig. 8-2.

- **Indirect pathway:** A second route linking the striatum with the GPi and
  SNr indirectly through the **GPe.** This **inhibitory pathway** increases the level
  of tonic inhibition (Fig. 8-2 and 8-3).

  - Cortical input to the striatum stimulates it to release GABA which inhib-
    its the **GPe** and prevents it from releasing more GABA. Decreased GABA
    levels release the STN from inhibition.

    - The STN is stimulated to release glutamate that activates the GPi.
    - The activated GPi releases GABA, which inhibits the thalamus
      (decreases motion).

## THE NIGROSTRIATAL PATHWAY

An important pathway in the modulation of the direct and indirect pathways
is the dopaminergic nigrostriatal projection from the SNpc to the striatum.

- Direct pathway striatal neurons have D1 dopamine receptors which
  depolarize the cell in response to dopamine and are stimulatory.

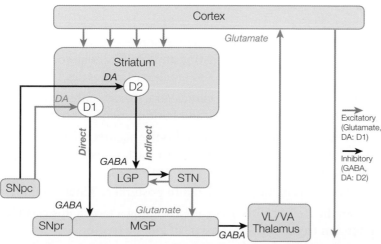

**FIGURE 8-2. Functional anatomy of the striatum.** Diagram of the main neurotransmitter
pathways and their effects in the cortical basal ganglia-thalamic circuits. Reproduced with
permission from Ropper AH, Brown *RH. Adams & Victor's Principles of Neurology, 8th ed.* New York:
McGraw-Hill, 2005.

**Functional Anatomy of Motor Cortex Basal Ganglia and Thalamus in Parkinson Disease**

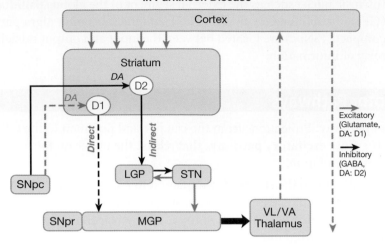

**FIGURE 8-3. Functional anatomy and Parkinson's disease.** Corresponding physiologic state as conceptualized in Parkinson's disease, in which hypokinesia is the main finding as a result of reduced dopamine input from the substantia nigra and pars compacta to the striatum via the direct pathway, which results in withdrawal of inhibitory activity of the globus pallidus and, in turn, increased inhibitory drive on the thalamic nuclei, which reduces input to the cortical motor system. Reproduced with permission from Ropper AH, Brown RH. *Adams & Victor's Principles of Neurology, 8th ed.* New York: McGraw-Hill, 2005.

## KEY FACT

**D1-R**eceptor: **DIR**ect

**In**direct: **In**hibitory

## KEY FACT

*Dopamine binds to D1-receptors, stimulating the excitatory pathway, and to D2-receptors, inhibiting the inhibitory pathway → Increases motion.*

- In contrast, indirect pathway striatal neurons have D2 dopamine receptors which hyperpolarize the cell in response to dopamine and are inhibitory.
- The nigrostriatal pathway thus has the dual effect of exciting the direct pathway while simultaneously inhibiting the indirect pathway.
- The loss of dopamine-producing neurons in the SNc causes paucity of movements that characterize Parkinson's disease.

## Types of Abnormal Movements

### TREMORS

- Tremor is the most common movement disorder encountered in clinical practice. Tremors consist of alternating and synchronous contractions of reciprocally innervated agonist and antagonistic muscles.
  - The most common tremors in clinical practice are enhanced physiological tremors, essential tremors (ET), and Parkinsonian rest tremors.
- The most important parameter assessed is the occurrence of tremor in relation to movement or position of a body part. Based on this, they are classified as rest or action tremors.
  - Action tremor is further classified into postural or kinetic tremor.
    - When the tremor worsens on approaching a target, it is classified as intention tremor, which is a type of kinetic tremor.
  - This distinction helps in identifying underlying pathophysiology and etiology, which in turn aids in the management.
- Tremor can also be classified based on its frequency, amplitude, anatomical distribution, exacerbating or alleviating factors, and associated neurological signs (Fig. 8-4).

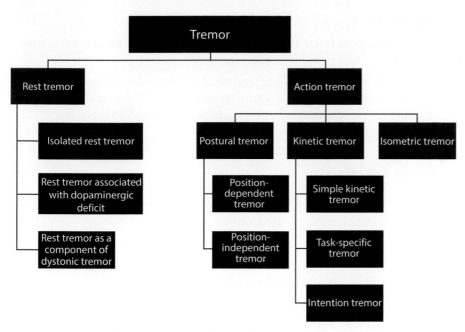

**FIGURE 8-4. Types of tremors.** From Lenka A, Jankovic J. *Tremor Syndromes: An Updated Review. Front Neurol.* 2021 Jul 26;12:684835.

■ **Resting tremors** are visible at rest and occur when a body part is completely supported against gravity. Resting tremors are minimal or absent during activity. They occur at a frequency of 3 to 6 Hz.

■ **Action tremors** are maximal when a body part is moved voluntarily. Action tremors may or may not change in severity as a target is reached; they can occur at very different frequencies, but the frequency is always <13 Hz. Action tremors include kinetic, intention, and postural tremors.

  • **Kinetic tremors** appear in the last part of a movement toward a target; amplitude is low.

  • **Intention tremors** occur during voluntary movement toward a target, but amplitude is high and frequency is low during the complete movement, while the tremor worsens as the target is reached (as seen in finger-to-nose testing). They occur at a frequency of 3 to 10 Hz.

  • **Postural tremors** are maximal when a limb is maintained in a fixed position against gravity (eg, holding the arms stretched out); they occur at a frequency of 5 to 8 Hz. Sometimes they are modified by specific positions or tasks, which may indicate their origin. For example, dystonia may trigger a tremor (dystonic tremor).

■ **Essential tremor (ET):**

  • ET is the **most common** tremor disorder. It is defined as a symmetric postural tremor with or without a kinetic component that involves hands and forearms, having a gradual onset, and should not be explained by any other underlying disorder.

  • Typically, ET is an action tremor, either postural or kinetic, that mainly affects the hands bilaterally with a frequency of 4 to 12 Hz.

    – The upper limbs are affected in about 95% of patients, followed by head (34%), lower limbs (20%), voice (12%), and trunk (5%).

    – In advanced cases, 20% to 30% of patients with ET may demonstrate resting tremor.

  • Family history is present but not necessary.

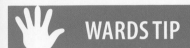
- Treatment:
  - The two most often-used drugs are nonselective β-blockers (eg, propranolol) and primidone (barbiturate).
  - In addition to the first-line treatments, many other drugs have been used as monotherapy or adjunctive treatment. Topiramate has been shown to be effective as well as gabapentin and alprazolam.
  - Improvement of essential tremor with alcohol is typical.

## RIGIDITY VS SPASTICITY

**Rigidity** and spasticity are two types of hypertonic states that are elicited when examining the muscle tone of extremities.

- Rigidity is a severe state of hypertonia where muscle resistance occurs throughout the entire range of motion of the affected joint.
  - Resistance is independent of velocity of movement.
  - It is frequently associated with lesions of the **basal ganglia.**
  - Individuals with rigidity present with stiffness, decreased range of motion, and loss of motor control.
- **Spasticity** is a condition in which muscles stiffen or tighten, preventing normal movement. The muscles remain contracted, and resist being stretched, thus affecting movement, speech, and gait.
  - Spasticity is caused by damage or disruption to the **nerve pathways within the brain or spinal cord** upper motor neurons that are responsible for controlling muscle and stretch reflexes.
  - These disruptions can be due to an imbalance in the inhibitory and excitatory signals sent to the muscles, causing them to lock in place.

## CHOREA

- Chorea is defined as involuntary, abrupt, and irregular movements that flow randomly from one part of the body to another.

| TABLE 8-1. Differences between Rigidity and Spasticity | |
|---|---|
| **Rigidity** | **Spasticity** |
| Increase in muscle tone due to damage to extrapyramidal pathways (basal ganglia) | Increase in muscle tone due to damage to the pyramidal tracts (commonest internal capsule) |
| Independent of velocity or amplitude of movement | Depends on velocity and amplitude of movement or stretch |
| Even detectable with slow movements | Best assessed by using rapid movements |
| Both flexors and extensors are affected | Mainly affects antigravity muscles |
| Movement resistance in both directions | Movement resistance in one direction (flexion or extension) |
| Can have associated static tremors | Absence of tremors |
| Typically, normo/hyporeflexia; no clonus | Can have associated hyperreflexia, clonus |
| Hypertonia—lead pipe (continuous) or cogwheel (interrupted) | Hypertonia—clasp knife (initial resistance followed by sudden release) |
| Example: Parkinson's disease | Example: hemiparesis (stroke), cerebral palsy, multiple sclerosis |

- It is often associated with an inability to sustain certain simple voluntary muscle contractions such as keeping eyes closed or protruding the tongue (called motor impersistence).
  - There are many causes of chorea. It is important to consider the age, acuity of onset, family history, associated symptoms, and the pattern and distribution of movements to determine the etiology. The different causes are summarized in Table 8-2.

Early symptoms may include simple clumsiness or incoordination.

- The most widely used agents in the treatment of chorea are *neuroleptics* due to their antidopaminergic activity.
  - Typical neuroleptics include haloperidol and fluphenazine.
  - Atypical neuroleptics include risperidone, olanzapine, clozapine, and quetiapine.

### TABLE 8-2. Various Causes of Chorea

| **Hereditary** |
| --- |
| Huntington's disease |
| Neuroacanthocytosis |
| Wilson's disease |
| **Drugs** |
| Neuroleptics |
| Antiepileptics (phenytoin, carbamazepine, valproate) |
| Stimulants (cocaine, amphetamines) |
| Others (Lithium, baclofen, phenothiazine) |
| **Toxins** |
| Alcohol |
| Anoxia |
| Carbon monoxide |
| Amphetamines, cocaine, heroin |
| Glue sniffing |
| Thallium, mercury |
| **Metabolic** |
| Hyponatremia, hypocalcemia, hypomagnesemia |
| Renal failure |
| Hyperthyroidism |
| Hyperglycemia and hypoglycemia |
| Hepatocerebral degeneration |
| **Immunologic** |
| SLE, antiphospholipid syndrome |
| Hashimoto's encephalopathy |
| Poststreptococcal (Sydenham chorea) |
| **Vascular** |
| Basal ganglia infarction or hemorrhage |

Source: Disorders of movement and posture. In: Ropper AH, Samuels MA, Klein JP, Prasad S, eds. *Adams and Victor's Principles of Neurology*, 11 ed. New York, NY: McGraw Hill; 2019: Table 4-4.

- Dopamine-depleting agents (eg, reserpine, tetrabenazine, deutetra-benazine) represent another option in the treatment of chorea.
- GABAergic drugs, such as clonazepam, gabapentin, and valproate, can be used as adjunctive therapy.

## DYSTONIA

- Dystonia is defined as a **sustained muscle contraction,** usually producing twisting, repetitive movements, or abnormal postures.
- Dystonia can be categorized in several ways:
  - Age of onset (young onset < 26 years or adult onset > 26 years).
  - Body distribution: focal (single area such as an arm), multifocal (noncontinuous body areas), generalized, or hemidystonia (one half of the body).
  - Etiology: Often classified as idiopathic dystonia or secondary dystonia. This distinction is important as it often influences management. Primary dystonias do not have other associated neurologic symptoms such as weakness, spasticity, ataxia, ocular motility abnormalities, retinal abnormalities, cognitive impairment, or seizures.
- The onset and progression of symptoms is gradual and without fixed postures unless there are contractures from long-standing dystonia.
- Secondary dystonia arises from an underlying associated condition.
  - Examples include a history of perinatal asphyxia or exposure to dopamine receptor antagonist drugs prior to development of dystonia.
- Blepharospasm is a common focal dystonia involving the periocular muscles.
  - Clinical manifestations: Increased blinking and spasms of involuntary eye closure.
  - Cervical dystonia (CD) affects the muscles of the neck and shoulders.
  - It may appear as horizontal turning of the head (torticollis), lateral flexion of the neck (laterocollis), forward flexion of the head (anterocollis), or posterior extension of the head (retrocollis).
- Treatment: symptomatic.
  - No curative therapies are available.
  - Oral medications for symptom control (tetrabenazine, clonazepam, baclofen).
  - Chemodenervation (injections of botulinum toxin).
  - Surgical management (reserved for patients with severe dystonia).
  - High-dose anticholinergic drugs have been of benefit in focal and generalized dystonia.

## HEMIBALLISMUS

The term comes from the Greek word *ballismos*, which means a jumping movement. The Latin word *ballista* refers to an ancient machine like a catapult used for flinging large stones. Hemiballismus, thus, refers to a neurologic syndrome of dramatic wild, flinging (forceful) movements occurring on one side of the body in an uninterrupted or continuous manner.

- The most common cause is a stroke (infarct or hemorrhage) of the contralateral subthalamic nucleus of the basal ganglia, resulting in disinhibition of the motor thalamus and cortex leading to contralateral hyperkinetic movements.
- Hyperglycemia can also cause hemiballismus.
- Treatment options include dopamine-depleting and dopamine-blocking agents.

## MYOCLONUS

Myoclonus refers to single or repetitive, brief, abrupt, jerky, asymmetric contractions involving parts of muscles or entire muscle/muscle groups. These are typically seen in the muscles of the extremities but can often be multifocal or diffuse. Myoclonus may also appear symmetrically on both sides of the body. Myoclonus can be classified in numerous ways, including the following:

- Epileptic vs nonepileptic
- Stimulus sensitive (reflex myoclonus) vs spontaneous
- Anatomic (peripheral, cortical, brainstem)
- Etiology: physiologic, essential, epileptic, symptomatic
- Antiepileptic drugs such as valproate, levetiracetam, and piracetam are effective in cortical myoclonus, but less effective in other forms of myoclonus.
- Clonazepam is typically helpful with all types of myoclonus.

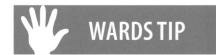

**WARDS TIP**

Myoclonus of the diaphragm is the cause of hiccups.

| TABLE 8-3. Causes of Myoclonus |
| --- |
| ***Epileptic forms*** |
| • Unverricht-Lundborg disease |
| • Lafora-body disease |
| • Baltic myoclonus |
| • Benign epilepsy with rolandic spikes |
| • Juvenile myoclonic epilepsy |
| • Infantile spasms (West syndrome) |
| • Cherry-red-spot myoclonus (sialidase deficiency) |
| • Myoclonus epilepsy with ragged red fibers (MERRF) |
| • Ceroid lipofuscinosis (Kufs disease) |
| • Tay-Sachs disease |
| • Epilepsia partialis continua |
| ***Essential forms*** |
| ***Myoclonic dementias*** |
| • Creutzfeldt-Jakob disease |
| • Subacute sclerosing panencephalitis |
| • Familial progressive poliodystrophy |
| • Alzheimer's, Lewy body, and Wilson's diseases (occasional in late stages) |
| • Whipple disease of the central nervous system |
| • Corticobasal ganglionic degeneration |
| • Dentatorubropallidoluysian atrophy |
| • AIDS dementia |

(Continued)

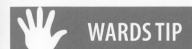

## WARDS TIP

Opsoclonus-myoclonus syndrome symptoms include rapid, repeated eye movements (opsoclonus) and repeated, brief muscle jerks in the arms and legs (myoclonus).

| TABLE 8-3. Causes of Myoclonus (Continued) |
| --- |
| ***Myoclonus with cerebellar disease (myoclonic ataxia)***<br>• Opsoclonus-myoclonus syndrome (paraneoplastic [anti-Ri], neuroblastoma, post- and parainfectious)<br>• Postanoxic myoclonus (Lance Adams type) |
| ***Metabolic, immune, and toxic disorders***<br>• Cerebral hypoxia (acute and severe)<br>• Uremia<br>• Hashimoto thyroiditis<br>• Lithium intoxication<br>• Haloperidol and sometimes phenothiazine intoxication<br>• Hepatic encephalopathy (rare)<br>• Cyclosporine toxicity<br>• Nicotinic acid deficiency encephalopathy<br>• Tetanus<br>• Other drug toxicities |
| ***Focal and spinal forms of myoclonus***<br>• Herpes zoster myelitis<br>• Other unspecified viral myelitis<br>• Multiple sclerosis<br>• Traumatic spinal cord injury<br>• Arteriovenous malformation of spinal cord<br>• Subacute myoclonic spinal neuronitis<br>• Paraneoplastic spinal myoclonus |

Source: Reproduced with permission from Disorders of movement and posture. In: Ropper AH, Samuels MA, Klein JP, Prasad S, eds. *Adams and Victor's Principles of Neurology, 11 ed.* New York, NY: McGraw Hill; 2019.

## ASTERIXIS

- Asterixis is a disorder of motor control characterized by an inability to actively maintain position and is thus a negative myoclonus.
  - Occurs when there is sudden, transient interruption or abnormal relaxation of ongoing muscle contraction, resulting in a brief loss of muscle tone in agonist muscles, followed by a compensatory jerk of the antagonistic muscles.
- **Bilateral** asterixis is usually due to metabolic encephalopathies or certain drugs, including phenytoin, valproate, carbamazepine, metoclopramide, and barbiturates.
  - Lithium can cause asterixis at both the therapeutic and toxic plasma levels.
- **Unilateral** asterixis is usually due to focal brain lesions in the genu and anterior portions of the internal capsule, ventrolateral thalamus, cerebellum, midbrain, and pons.
  - Common in hepatic diseases, and less commonly due to azotemia, metabolic derangements, and respiratory disease.
  - Tested by extending the arms, dorsiflexing the wrists, and spreading the fingers to observe for the "flap" at the wrist.

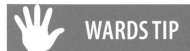

## WARDS TIP

Bilateral asterixis is most commonly associated with metabolic encephalopathies, especially hepatic.

## WARDS TIP

Unilateral asterixis is often due to focal brain lesions in the thalamus

## Selected Movement Disorders

### IDIOPATHIC PARKINSON'S DISEASE

Idiopathic Parkinson's disease (PD) is a chronic, progressive, and disabling neurodegenerative disorder characterized by both motor and non-motor symptoms. This is typically caused by a loss of the predominately dopamine-producing neurons in the substantia nigra of the midbrain. PD is a heterogeneous disorder characterized by various clinical presentations, age of onset, types of nonmotor symptoms, and different rates of progression. While some patients have a relatively benign disease course with favorable response to dopaminergic therapy, others appear to progress more rapidly.

*Pathology*

- PD is characterized by the loss of dopaminergic neurons in the nigrostriatal system and the accumulation of Lewy bodies (alpha synuclein) in the midbrain.
  - Motor symptoms become evident when 60% to 80% of dopaminergic neurons are lost in the pars compacta of the substantia nigra.
- The cause of PD is unknown, with both inherited and environmental factors being believed to play a role in the deterioration of dopaminergic neurons.
- Those with a family history of PD are at an increased risk.
  - Most cases are sporadic, although several genes have been implicated in familial forms of PD.
  - It is estimated that 5% to 10% of patients have a genetic etiology for the disease. Monogenic forms of PD include mutations in the PARK gene among others.
  - Exposure to pesticides, metals, solvents, and other toxins has been studied. No definitive causal relationship has been established yet.

*Clinical Symptoms/Diagnosis*

- PD is a clinical diagnosis. Asymmetric symptoms of resting tremor, bradykinesia, and rigidity with favorable response to dopaminergic therapy suggest its diagnosis.
- Exclusionary features may include severe dysautonomia, early hallucinations, dementia preceding motor symptoms, and postural instability and freezing within the first 3 years after diagnosis.

**Clinical diagnostic criteria:**

- Bradykinesia (slow initiation of voluntary movement with progressive reduction in speed and amplitude of repetitive actions)
- And at least one of the following:
  - Muscle rigidity
  - Resting tremor
  - Postural instability (not caused by primary visual, vestibular, cerebellar, or proprioceptive dysfunction)

**Supportive criteria:**

- Three or more required for definitive diagnosis.

**Nonmotor symptoms:**

- Cognitive/Behavioral: mood changes, hallucinations, psychosis, compulsive behaviors, dementia late in the disease course
- Autonomic: orthostatic hypotension, constipation, delayed gastric emptying, sialorrhea, urinary and sexual dysfunction, hyposmia
- Sleep/REM sleep behavioral disorder
- Speech and swallowing changes

**Neuroimaging of PD:**

- PD is a clinical diagnosis. However, neuroimaging technology such as the dopamine transporter single-photon emission computed tomography

## KEY FACT

- Unilateral onset
- Resting tremor
- Progressive symptoms
- Persistent asymmetry
- Excellent response to Levodopa
- Severe Levodopa-induced chorea
- Levodopa response for 5 years or more
- Clinical course of 10 years or more

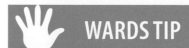

## WARDS TIP

**Parkinson's "TRAPS" a patient.**

T   tremors at rest
R   rigidity
A   akinesia (or bradykinesia)
P   postural instability
S   shuffling gait

(SPECT) scan may be helpful in making a diagnosis, especially in clinically ambiguous presentations.

- Dopamine transporter SPECT is not a confirmatory test for PD, nor is it intended to differentiate between PD and other degenerative forms of Parkinsonism, including atypical Parkinsonism. Clinicians may decide to order a dopamine transporter SPECT when the diagnosis of a clinical tremor syndrome is uncertain (eg, when differentiating between PD tremor and ET).

*Treatment: Categories of Medications in PD (Fig. 8-5)*

### Increase L-DOPA availability:

- These agents prevent peripheral (pre-BBB) L-DOPA degradation, thus increasing the amount of L-DOPA entering the CNS. This increases the central L-DOPA available for conversion to dopamine.
  - Levodopa/Carbidopa: Carbidopa blocks the peripheral conversion of L-DOPA by blocking DOPA carboxylase (DDC).
  - Entacapone and tolcapone prevent peripheral breakdown of L-DOPA to 3-O-methyldopa (3-OMD) by blocking COMT (catechol-O-methyltransferase).

### Dopamine agonists:

- These agents directly bind to postsynaptic receptors to stimulate dopamine release.
  - Bromocriptine (ergot)
  - Pramipexole, ropinirole (non-ergot)

### Prevent dopamine breakdown in glial cells:

- These agents act centrally (post-BBB) to inhibit breakdown of dopamine within the glial cells.
  - MAO-B inhibitors: Selegeline, rasageline
  - COMT inhibitors: Entocapone, Tolcapone

### Increase dopamine availability:

- Amantadine is an anti-viral agent.
  - Mechanism of action in PD is poorly understood. However, it is thought to increase the dopamine availability through multiple mechanisms: preventing dopamine reuptake, facilitating presynaptic dopamine release, and blocking glutamate NMDA receptors.

### Curb excess cholinergic activity:

- These agents are typically antimuscarinic agents that improve tremors and rigidity, but have little effect on bradykinesia.
  - Benztropine
  - Biperidine
  - Procyclidine
  - Trihexphenidyl

## ATYPICAL PARKINSONIAN SYNDROMES

The atypical Parkinsonian syndromes are synucleinopathies and tauopathies, that is, disorders characterized by the abnormal deposition of the proteins α-synuclein and tau. The site of deposition is correlated with the clinical features. These syndromes include dementia with Lewy bodies (DLB), multiple

**KEY FACT**

*Entacapone only acts peripherally (pre-BBB) to prevent peripheral L-DOPA degradation, thus increasing the amount of L-DOPA entering the CNS.*

| DRUGS COMMONLY USED IN THE TREATMENT OF PARKINSON DISEASE | | | | |
|---|---|---|---|---|
| MEDICATION | STARTING DOSE | TARGET DOSE | MAIN BENEFIT | SIDE EFFECTS |
| **L-Dopa** | | | | |
| Carbidopa-L-dopa | 25/100 mg tid | Up to 50/250 mg q3h | Reduction of tremor and bradykinesia; less effect on postural difficulties | Nausea, dyskinesias, orthostatic hypotension, hallucinations, confusion |
| Controlled release carbidopa-L-dopa | 25/100 mg tid | Up to 50/200 mg q4h | May prolong L-dopa effects | |
| **Dopamine agonists** | | | | |
| Ropinirole | 0.25 mg tid | 9-24 mg/d | Moderate effects on all aspects; reduced motor fluctuations of L-dopa | Orthostatic hypotension, excessive and abrupt sleepiness, confusion, hallucinations |
| Pramipexole | 0.125 mg tid | 0.75-3 mg/d | As above | |
| **Glutamate antagonist** | | | | |
| Amantadine | 100 mg/d | 100 mg bid–tid | Smoothing of motor fluctuations | Leg swelling, congestive heart failure, prostatic outlet obstruction, confusion, hallucinations, insomnia |
| **Anticholinergics** | | | | |
| Benztropine | 0.5 mg/d | Up to 4 mg/d | Tremor reduction, less effect on other features | Atropinic effects: dry mouth, urinary outlet obstruction, confusion, and psychosis |
| Trihexyphenidyl | 0.5 mg bid | Up to 2 mg tid | As above | As above |
| **COMT inhibitors** | | | | |
| Entacapone | 200 mg with L-dopa | | Prolonged effect of L-dopa | Urine discoloration, diarrhea, increased dyskinesias |
| **MAO-inhibitors** | | | | |
| Rasagiline | 0.5 mg | 1 mg daily | Reduced "off" time, potential neuroprotection | Hypertensive crisis with tyramine-rich foods and sympathomimetics |
| Selegiline | 5 mg | 5 mg bid | Potential neuroprotection | |

**FIGURE 8-5. Parkinson's disease medications and their mechanisms of action**. Reproduced, with permission, from Degenerative diseases of the nervous system. In: Ropper AH, Samuels MA, Klein JP, Prasad S, eds. *Adams and Victor's Principles of Neurology*, 11th ed. New York, NY: McGraw Hill; 2019: Table 38-4.

system atrophy (MSA), progressive supranuclear palsy (PSP), and corticobasal degeneration (CBD).

■ In DLB, synuclein is mainly deposited in neocortical neurons, with some brainstem involvement. The main clinical features are dementia and, later on, Parkinsonism.

■ In MSA, synuclein is deposited in oligodendrocytes, mainly in the cerebellum but also in the brainstem. The main clinical feature is autonomic dysfunction combined with Parkinsonism or cerebellar ataxia.

■ Synucleinopathies often impair REM (rapid eye movement) sleep.

■ PSP and CBD, on the other hand, are primary tauopathies.

• PSP causes predominantly supranuclear vertical gaze palsy and early postural instability with falls.

• CBD manifests as markedly asymmetrical Parkinsonism with apraxia or cortical sensory disturbance.

■ At present, there is no accepted treatment for any of these disorders; the available symptomatic treatments are of limited efficacy and are supported only by low-level evidence.

*Multiple System Atrophy (MSA)*

■ MSA is an adult-onset neurodegenerative disorder that is clinically characterized by various combinations of Parkinsonism, cerebellar, autonomic, and motor dysfunction.

- Together with PD and DLB, MSA belongs to the group of α-synucleinopathies, which are characterized by abnormal accumulation of fibrillary alpha synuclein.

- MSA specifically involves the nigrostriatal, olivopontocerebellar, and autonomic nervous systems.

- MSA is characterized clinically by symptoms that can be subdivided into pyramidal, extrapyramidal, cerebellar, and autonomic categories.

  - Extrapyramidal motor abnormalities such as bradykinesia, rigidity, and postural instability are classified as either Parkinsonian-type (MSA-P) or cerebellar (MSA-C).

  - Additionally, MSA patients develop behavioral alterations such as depression and executive dysfunction that suggest frontal lobe impairment.

  - Autonomic dysfunction may be the only presenting feature in some MSA patients.

    - Severe **orthostatic hypotension** is the main symptom of cardiovascular autonomic failure, often manifested as recurrent syncope, dizziness, nausea, headache, and weakness.

    - Orthostatic hypotension usually occurs after the onset of genitourinary symptoms.

    - Other nonmotor features include constipation, vasomotor failure with diminished sweating (hypohydrosis), pupillomotor abnormalities, and oculomotor dysfunctions.

- MRI abnormalities include:

  - "**Hot cross bun**" sign—a cruciform hyperintensity in the pons (Fig. 8-6).

  - Current therapeutic interventions for MSA are aimed at the treatment of symptoms such as hypotension, erectile dysfunction, and gastrointestinal dysfunction, rather than at the underlying pathology itself.

    - There are no causative or disease-modifying treatments available and symptomatic therapies are limited.

    - Levodopa responsiveness has been reported initially in some MSA-P patients, but the effect is usually transient.

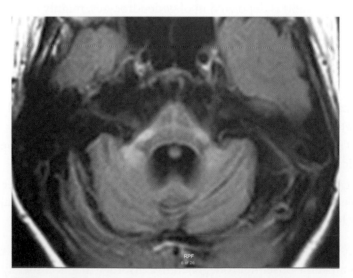

**FIGURE 8-6. MRI in multiple system atrophy.** Axial FLAIR MRI demonstrating the "hot cross bun" sign and middle cerebellar peduncle atrophy in a patient with MSA-C. Reproduced, with permission, from Berkowitz AL. *Clinical Neurology and Neuroanatomy: A Localization-Based Approach.* New York, NY: McGraw Hill; 2017: Figure 23-3.

*Progressive Supranuclear Palsy (PSP)*

- PSP is a form of atypical Parkinsonian syndrome that can affect movement, gait, balance, speech, swallowing, vision, eye movements, mood, behavior, and cognition. PSP is an akinetic-rigid form of Parkinsonism.

- The defining histopathologic feature of PSP is an intracerebral aggregation of the microtubule-associated protein tau.

- Early in the course of the disease, motor abnormalities are typically axial. Gait difficulty and **falls** are the most common initial manifestation.

  - As the disease progresses, other neurologic manifestations occur, including worsening Parkinsonism, dysarthria, dysphagia, frontal cognitive difficulties, and eye movement abnormalities.

  - Although **supranuclear ophthalmoplegia** is the hallmark of PSP, some patients only manifest this late in the progression of the disease.

  - Typically, downgaze is impaired before the upgaze.

- Neuroimaging in patients with PSP by MRI:

  - Atrophy and signal increase in the midbrain, degeneration of the red nucleus, atrophy of the pons and cerebellum, and signal increase in the inferior olives.

  - The "**hummingbird sign**" is often present, in which the shape of the rostral midbrain atrophy on midsagittal images looks like a hummingbird (Fig. 8-7).

- The treatment remains symptomatic and supportive.

  - For motor (Parkinsonian) symptoms, levodopa combined with a dopa decarboxylase inhibitor (eg, carbidopa) can be tried, often with modest to no success.

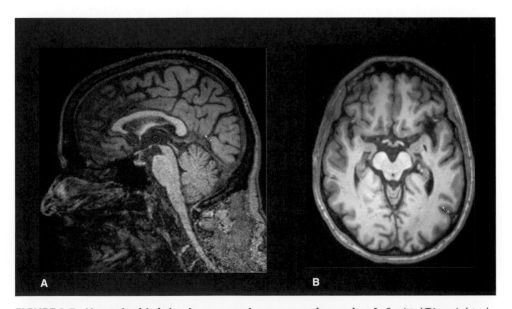

**FIGURE 8-7. Hummingbird sign in progressive supranuclear palsy. A.** Sagittal T1-weighted MRI demonstrating the hummingbird sign (midbrain atrophy with spared pons). **B.** Axial T1-weighted MRI demonstrating the Mickey Mouse sign (decreased anteroposterior size of the midbrain when measured from between the cerebral peduncles to the superior colliculi, leading to a "carved out" appearance between the cerebral peduncles). Reproduced, with permission, from Berkowitz AL. *Clinical Neurology and Neuroanatomy: A Localization-Based Approach.* New York, NY: McGraw Hill; 2017: Figure 23-4.

*Corticobasal Degeneration (CBD)*

- CBD is a rare neurodegenerative disorder involving the cerebral cortex and basal ganglia. It results in marked disorders in movement and cognition and is classified as one of the Parkinson plus syndromes.
  - Characterized by akinetic-rigid Parkinsonism, dystonic and myoclonic movements.
  - Associated with cortical symptoms such as ideomotor apraxia, alien limb phenomena, aphasia, or sensory neglect.
  - Deficits in language and visuospatial dysfunction are also characteristic in addition to cognitive changes. In some cases, language dysfunction is the first symptom.
- Three distinct phenotypes: corticobasal syndrome (CBS), frontal behavioral-spatial syndrome (FBS), and nonfluent/agrammatic variant of primary progressive aphasia (naPPA).

## HUNTINGTON'S DISEASE (HD)

Huntington's disease (HD), a neurodegenerative autosomal-dominant disorder, is characterized by involuntary choreoathetotic movements with cognitive and behavioral disturbances. HD results from degeneration of neurons in the putamen, caudate, and the cerebral cortex.

- Cytosine, adenine, and guanine (CAG) trinucleotide repeats on the short arm of chromosome 4p in the Huntingtin (HTT) gene. This leads to an abnormally long expansion of the polyglutamine in the HTT protein, which leads to neurodegeneration.

The anticipation phenomenon is seen in the paternal line of inheritance, which arises due to the instability of the CAG repeats during spermatogenesis. Anticipation leads to a phenomenon where an affected offspring of a patient with the condition will develop the disorder at a younger age than the relative who passed on that gene. HD commonly affects patients between the ages of 30 and 50 years. However, the longer the CAG repeats, the earlier the onset of symptoms.

- The signs and symptoms classically consist of motor, cognitive, and psychiatric disturbances.
  - Other less common features include weight loss, sleep disturbances, and autonomic nervous system dysfunction.
  - Motor symptoms include the characteristic unwanted involuntary choreiform movements which initially begin in the distal extremities but could go on to affect the facial muscles as well. In later stages, however, bradykinesia and dystonia predominate.
- Diagnosis can be made clinically in a patient with motor and/or cognitive and behavioral disturbances with a parent diagnosed with HD and confirmed by DNA testing.
  - DNA testing is the gold standard and is also used to quantify the size of the CAG repeat.
- MRI findings are present before overt clinical manifestation (Fig. 8-8).
  - Adult onset of HD is typically characterized by early atrophy in the caudate.
  - Cerebellar and cortical atrophy are seen later in the disease.
- No cure for the disease, and affected patients tend to be entirely dependent on their caregiver as the disease progresses. Therefore, treatment is aimed at improving the quality of life and decreasing complications.

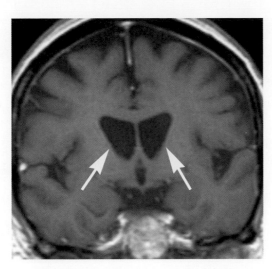

**FIGURE 8-8. Caudate atrophy with ex-vacuo dilation of the lateral ventricles in Huntington's disease.** Image demonstrates enlarged frontal horns with flattened edge due to caudate atrophy (*arrows*) with abnormal configuration. Reproduced, with permission, from Jameson J, Fauci AS, Kasper DL, et al. *Harrison's Principles of Internal Medicine*, 20th ed. New York, NY: McGraw Hill; 2018.

- The American Academy of Neurology guidelines recommends the use of tetrabenazine (TBZ), amantadine, or riluzole in managing chorea.

## WILSON'S DISEASE

- Wilson's disease or hepatolenticular degeneration is an **autosomal recessive** disease which results in **excess copper** build-up, primarily affecting the liver and basal ganglia of the brain.

- The genetic defect is localized to long arm of chromosome 13 (13q) at the Wilson's Disease protein (ATP7B) gene, which has been shown to alter the copper transporting ATP gene in the liver.

- The majority of patients with Wilson's disease present within the first decade of life with **liver dysfunction**.

  - Neuropsychiatric features are seen in the third/fourth decade of life in about 30% to 50% of patients.

    - Symptoms include hyperkinetic and hypokinetic movements (tremors, chorea, hemiballismus), muscle stiffness, trouble speaking, mood and personality changes, anxiety, and auditory or visual hallucinations.

  - Liver-related symptoms include vomiting, weakness, ascites, peripheral edema, abdominal pain, jaundice, and itchiness.

- On physical exam, the patient may have features of **hepatosplenomegaly**, isolated splenomegaly, or if the disease has progressed to cirrhosis, stigmata of chronic liver disease.

  - An eye exam may reveal icterus of sclerae and slit-lamp examination for **Kayser-Fleischer (KF)** ring (Fig. 8-9) which is a golden brown discoloration around the cornea (*note that the only other disorder with KF rings is primary biliary cirrhosis*).

- Laboratory findings include increased serum copper and **reduced serum ceruloplasmin**

  - Increased 24-hour urinary copper excretion is the most sensitive screening test.

- Treatment consists of copper chelation with D-penicillamine, trientine in conjunction with zinc.

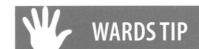

**WARDS TIP**

"Wing-beating" tremor is typical of Wilson's disease. It is characterized by a low-frequency, high-amplitude, posture-induced proximal arm tremor, elicited by sustained abduction of the arms, with flexed elbows and palms facing downward.

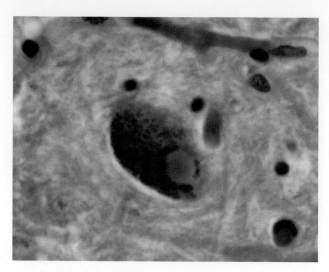

**FIGURE 8-9. Kayser-Fleischer rings in Wilson's disease.** Reproduced with permission from Allan H. Ropper, Martin A. Samuels, Joshua P. Klein, Sashank Prasad, *Adams and Victor's Principles of Neurology, 11e*, figure 38.5. ISBN 978007 1842617. From Frosch MP, et al: The central nervous system. In Robbins SL, et al (eds): *Robbins and Cotran Pathologic Basis of Disease, 8th ed*. Philadelphia, Saunders/Elsevier, 2010.

## DRUG-INDUCED MOVEMENT DISORDERS

Drug-induced movement disorders (DIMDs), also commonly referred to as extrapyramidal symptoms (EPS), represent a variety of iatrogenic and clinically distinct movement disorders, including akathisia, tardive dyskinesia, tremors, acute dystonic reaction, and drug-induced Parkinsonism. These are typically seen with the use of dopamine-blocking or dopamine-receptor blocking agents.

### *Akathisia*

■ Akathisia comes from a Greek word *a-kathízein*, meaning "not to sit." It is a combination of subjective inner restlessness/agitation and a compelling need to move, rock, or pace but movements do not bring relief.

■ It is a well-recognized side effect of antipsychotic and antiemetic drugs but may also be caused by other widely prescribed drugs.

■ On diagnosis, the offending or suspected drug should be withdrawn or the dose reduced if possible.

■ Where this is not possible, propranolol or other lipophilic β-blockers are the most effective. Benzodiazepines can be considered as additional treatment.

### *Tardive Dyskinesia (TD)*

■ The term *dyskinesia* refers to involuntary muscle movements that can range from slight tremor to uncontrollable movement of the entire body.

• TD gets its name from the slow—or tardive—onset of involuntary movements of the face, lips, tongue, trunk, and extremities.

■ TD most generally occurs in individuals who are on long-term treatment with dopaminergic antagonist medications (antipsychotic drugs [APDs]).

• These include first- and second-generation neuroleptics, certain antidepressants (fluoxetine), lithium, and some antiemetics (metoclopramide, especially in older individuals), and antihistamines.

■ Prevention is the mainstay of management.

• Dopamine receptor antagonists should be avoided whenever possible by selecting other medications that have a lower potential to cause tardive dyskinesia.

- Chronic use of first-generation antipsychotics should be avoided whenever possible.
  - Treatment options include clonazepam.
    - Valbenazine, a vesicular monoamine transport type 2 (VMAT2) inhibitor, is also FDA approved for the treatment of tardive dyskinesia.

## Ataxia and Gait Abnormalities

**Ataxia** is a neurological sign that manifests in a lack of coordination in the movement of different muscles in the body. It is a clinical finding, not a disease.

- It results from dysfunction of the brain areas responsible for the coordination of movements, most commonly the cerebellum.
- The three types of ataxia, according to the location, are cerebellar, sensory, and vestibular.
  - Ataxia can also subdivide into **sporadic** (patients have no family history of ataxia and manifesting in adulthood), **hereditary** (caused by a defect in a gene and manifesting in childhood), and **acquired** (due to structural or demyelinating conditions, toxicity, paraneoplastic, inflammatory or infections, and autoimmune conditions).
    - **Friedreich ataxia** is an autosomal recessive form of ataxia and the commonest among the hereditary forms.

Ataxia may occur due to abnormalities in different areas of the nervous system, including the brain, spinal cord, nerves, and nerve roots. Common etiologies are as follows:

- Focal lesions—due to tumors, stroke, multiple sclerosis, or inflammation
- Metabolic—due to substances such as alcohol, antidepressant drugs, and antiepileptic drugs
- Radiation
- Vitamin B12 deficiency
- Thyroid disease—hypothyroidism
- Head injury
- Celiac disease (gluten ataxia)
- Hereditary—Friedreich ataxia, ataxia-telangiectasia, Niemann-Pick disease, fragile X associated ataxia/tremor syndrome
- Arnold-Chiari malformation
- Wilson's disease

## WORK UP OF ATAXIAS

- Depending on the location of the lesion, characteristic findings are as follows:
  1. Lesions in the lateral cerebellum cause symptoms on the same side as the lesion (ipsilateral).
  2. Lesions in the cerebellum hemisphere cause limb ataxia.
  3. Lesions in the vermis cause truncal, gait ataxia with sparing of the limbs.
  4. Lesions at vestibulocerebellar areas cause disbalance, vertigo, and gait ataxia.

The selection of tests necessary to make the diagnosis are guided by clinical presentation and clinical suspicion.

- Blood tests for specific deficiencies, drugs, and toxins may be in order.
- Urinalysis can look for mercury level measurement.
- Brain imaging includes a CT scan as an initial study, but MRI is critical to visualize structural lesions, strokes, and congenital or acquired abnormalities.
  - Imaging of the spinal cord with MRI is indicated if a spine lesion is suspected.
- Genetic testing is the diagnostic course for inherited ataxias.

## GAIT DISORDERS

- Are described as any deviation from normal walking or gait.
- Numerous diseases affect both the central and peripheral nervous systems, which ultimately affect gait.
- Sensory ataxia caused by polyneuropathy, subcortical vascular encephalopathy, or dementia is among the most common neurological causes.
- Neurodegenerative disorders including Parkinson's, Huntington's, and normal pressure hydrocephalus can alter cognitive functions to the point that walking can become a difficult task.
- Weakness of the hip and lower extremity muscles commonly cause gait disturbances.
- Cerebral palsy, muscular dystrophy, Charcot Marie Tooth disease, ataxia-telangiectasia, spinal muscular atrophy, peroneal neuropathy, and white-matter disease all cause significant gait disabilities.

The examination can separate gait disturbances into two categories: musculoskeletal or neuromuscular (lower motor neuron and upper motor neuron).

- **Trendelenburg gait:** pelvis drops to the unaffected side
  - Cause: hip abductor weakness
- Steppage gait: unable to heel strike causing initial contact with toes (foot drop)
  - Cause: ankle dorsiflexion weakness
- **Waddling gait:** toe walking (posterior lurch and bilateral Trendelenburg)
  - Cause: proximal muscle weakness
- **Scissor gait** cerebral palsy
  - Cause: prolonged neonatal hypoxia, brain injury during birth
- **Ataxic gait:** broad-based, unsteady
  - Cause: cerebellar syndrome (alcohol, phenytoin, stroke, tumor, degenerative, inflammatory)
- **Sensory ataxic gait** (stomping gait): Romberg's test positive. Vitamin B12 deficiency. The patients use visual control to compensate for the loss of proprioception
- **Hemiparetic gait** (hemispastic): gait is slow with a broad base with both knee and hip extended; during the swing phase, the paretic leg performs a lateral movement (circumduction)
  - **Cause:** stroke, tumor, trauma, degenerative, inflammatory, vasculitis

- **Festinating gait** (Shuffling gait): short stepped, hurrying, with weak arm swing, or naturally very slow (Parkinsonian).
  - Cause: Parkinson's disease
- **Apraxic frontal gait:** gait ignition failure, or with walking difficulty ("Marche à petit pas"). Bifrontal lesions
- **Magnetic gait:** slow gait with unsteady turns, broad-based, short-stepped; "stuck to the floor," or "glued to the floor" words are often used
  - Cause: normal pressure hydrocephalus (NPH)

## TICS

- Tics are sudden, stereotyped, repetitive movements or vocalization that may look intentional but serve no useful purpose.
  - Patients often describe a compelling urge to perform the movement/ vocalization and may be able to suppress the movement transiently.
    - Suppression builds up inner tension which is relieved by the movement or vocalization.
    - May be exacerbated by stress or anxiety and can be relieved by distraction.
- Tics almost always begin in childhood, most often ages 3 to 10 years, and on average, tics are most severe around ages 9 to 11.
- Chronic tic disorders are defined by the persistence of tics for at least 12 months.
- **Tourette's Disorder (TS):** Childhood onset of idiopathic chronic tics characterized by both movement and vocalization.
  - TS is a genetic disorder.
  - Often times, TS is associated with learning disability and obsessive-compulsive disorder (OCD).
  - The tics may change over time.
- **Persistent (Chronic) Motor Tic Disorder (CTD):** Tics are only motor movements (without vocalization).

Tics are classified as simple or complex.

- Simple motor tics include forceful blinking, raising the eyebrows, turning the head, shrugging, or sniffing.
- Simple vocal tics involve sounds made by moving air through the nose or mouth, including grunting, hissing, snorting, throat clearing.
- Complex motor tics can be a combination of many simple motor tics or a series of movements that involve more than one muscle group. These types of tics can interfere greatly with daily life and may be harmful.
  - Examples include head banging, lip biting, spitting, finger cracking, gyrating movements, facial grimacing.
- Complex vocal tics may involve words, phrases, and sentences. Patients with a complex vocal tic may repeat their own words (**palilalia**) or other people's words (**echolalia**) and may use obscene words (**coprolalia**).

In most cases, motor and vocal tics are not dangerous or disruptive to a person's everyday life and no treatment is necessary.

- For those with severe tics that interfere with quality of life, tics may be managed with medications that include neuroleptics and other sedatives.
- Specific psychiatric medications or psychotherapy may be needed in cases of Obsessive-compulsive disorder (OCD)

**Case 1:** A 67-year-old man is seen by the physician because of a 1-year history of difficulty sleeping. After he gets into bed at night, his legs feel cold and crampy, and he cannot settle into a comfortable position. Walking around temporarily relieves the symptoms. He also has difficulty sitting for prolonged periods of time. Vital signs are within normal limits. Examination shows no abnormalities. Which of the following is the most likely diagnosis?

A. Benign fasciculations
B. Major depressive disorder
C. Parkinson's disease
D. REM sleep behavior disorder
E. Restless legs syndrome

The correct answer is E. This patient presents with symptoms of cold and crampy legs, consistent with Restless legs syndrome, which typically occur at bedtime and improve with walking.

**Case 2:** An 84-year-old man has noticed tremor and stiffness of the right hand over the past 3 months. On examination, the tremor disappears when he reaches to grab a pen. Movements are slower on the right than the left, including his walking speed. He has cogwheel rigidity of the right arm and diminished blink rate. His voice is also faint and speech is slow. What is the standard medication for this condition?

A. Carbidopa-levodopa
B. Haldol
C. Sertraline
D. Rivastigmine
E. Methylphenidate

The correct answer is A. The patient exhibits signs and symptoms of idiopathic Parkinson's disease. The treatment is carbidopa-levodopa.

**Case 3:** A 34-year-old man develops depression and memory problems over a 6-month period. His initial neurological evaluation reveals a metabolic acidosis associated with his dementia. His liver is firm. He has tremor and rigidity in his arms and walks with relatively little swing in his arms. His blink is substantially reduced, which gives him the appearance of staring. With sustained abduction of the arms, with flexed elbows and palms facing downward, there is a low-frequency, high-amplitude, posture-induced proximal arm tremor. What is the diagnosis?

A. Huntington's disease
B. Alzheimer's disease
C. Wilson's disease
D. Behçet's disease
E. Conversion disorder

The correct answer is C. The tremor observed is the so-called "wing-beating" tremor typical of Wilson's disease. The metabolic acidosis, firm liver, depression, and Parkinsonism are part of the constellation of symptoms due to copper deposits throughout the body. One other key sign is the Kayser-Fleischer rings observed in the cornea.

In this chapter, we review the main neuromuscular topics that will be seen in clinic, on the wards, and on the shelf exam. We will focus on diseases of peripheral nerves, the neuromuscular junction, and skeletal muscle itself. It will be important to keep in mind the classic presentation of each, as well as localization, differential diagnosis, workup, and treatment.

## Types of Neuropathies

### DISTAL SYMMETRIC SENSORY POLYNEUROPATHIES

Distal symmetric sensory polyneuropathies are length-dependent, with symptoms beginning in the feet. Some include autonomic involvement (cardiovascular, GI, GU, skin, visual, or thermoregulatory symptoms) such as diabetes and amyloidosis.

- Differential diagnosis
  - Diabetes (30%)
  - Alcohol (30%)
  - Idiopathic etiologies (30%)
  - Less commonly: Amyloidosis, and vitamin B1 or B12 deficiencies.
- Diagnostics
  - Hemoglobin A1c
  - Thyroid Function Test
  - Vitamin B12, homocysteine, methylmalonic acid
  - EMG/Nerve Conduction Study
  - Serum protein electrophoresis and immunofixation

### DIFFUSE MOTOR NEUROPATHIES

Diffuse motor neuropathies result in symmetric weakness and hyporeflexia.

- Diagnostics
  - EMG/NCS to assess for demyelination
  - CSF (cells and protein)
- Differential diagnosis
  - Acute inflammatory demyelinating polyneuropathy (AIDP) and Guillain-Barre syndrome (GBS)
    - Can also include autonomic involvement
  - Diphtheria
  - Chronic inflammatory demyelinating polyneuropathy (CIDP)
    - Can also include autonomic involvement
  - Osteosclerotic myeloma
  - Inherited: Charcot-Marie-Tooth disease, Spinal Muscular Atrophy, familial Amyotrophic Lateral Sclerosis, Kennedy Disease
  - Acute Intermittent Porphyria
  - Drugs (amiodarone, perhexiline, gold)
  - Acute Arsenic

---

**WARDS TIP**

Lesion in brain or spinal cord causes upper motor neuron sign of hyper-reflexia. Lesion of nerve roots or peripheral nerves causes lower motor neuron sign of hypo-reflexia.

## MULTIFOCAL MOTOR AND SENSORY NEUROPATHIES

Multifocal motor and sensory neuropathies result in asymmetric weakness and sensory deficits.

- Differential diagnosis
  - Immune-mediated
    - Vasculitis, sarcoidosis
  - Infectious
    - Lyme disease, CMV, Leprosy, Herpes Zoster
  - Infiltrative
    - Diabetic amyotrophy, amyloid, lymphomatous infiltration
  - Hereditary
  - Charcot-Marie-Tooth X
  - Hereditary neuropathy with liability to pressure palsies (HNPP)

## IMMUNE-MEDIATED NEUROPATHIES

*Guillain-Barre Syndrome (GBS) or Acute Inflammatory Demyelinating Polyradiculopathy (AIDP)*

- Epidemiology: Highest incidence in adulthood. Not seen in infants
- Signs and symptoms
  - Initially back pain and paresthesias
  - **Ascending, bilateral flaccid paralysis** following stocking-glove distribution
  - **Hyporeflexia/areflexia**, mild tingling/numbness
  - Respiratory insufficiency or failure
  - Autonomic instability (ie, brady/tachycardia, sweating, pupillary changes, orthostasis)
  - Liver function enzyme changes
  - Less than 4 weeks of symptoms (if lasting over 4 weeks, consider CIDP)
- Pathophysiology
  - Commonly follow an illness, trauma, or vaccination in prior month
  - T-cell autoimmunity, cross-reactive autoantibodies attack host axonal antigens
  - Occasionally autoantibodies against *Campylobacter jejuni*, CMV, EBV, mycoplasma
- Diagnostics
  - CSF demonstrates **albuminocytologic dissociation** (high protein with normal cell count), especially after 2 weeks
  - Nerve conduction study: Demyelinating findings
  - MRI: Nerve root enhancement
- Treatment
  - Secure airway and monitor respiratory status. Consider ICU monitoring and intubation
  - Symptomatic treatment of autonomic instability
  - IVIG or plasmapheresis
  - Do NOT treat with corticosteroids (not shown to improve outcomes)

*Chronic Inflammatory Demyelinating Polyneuropathy (CIDP)*

- Signs and symptoms
  - Diffuse, symmetric weakness, and hyporeflexia developing over 8 weeks or more
  - Time course can be relapsing-remitting, monophasic, or chronically progressive
  - Associated with autoimmune disorders (diabetes), malignancies (lymphoma, leukemia, hepatocellular carcinoma), infections (HIV)
  - Good prognosis, but high relapse rate
- Treatment
  - Corticosteroids (ie, oral prednisone)
  - IVIG, plasma exchange, cyclosporine, azathioprine
  - Cyclophosphamide for refractory cases

*Multifocal Motor Neuropathy (MMN)*

- Epidemiology: Mostly affects >40 years old, males more than females
- Signs and symptoms
  - Cramps and fasciculations which lead to focal weakness (ie, wrist drop, intrinsic hand weakness, foot drop)
  - Slowly progressive
- Diagnostics
  - **Anti-GM1** antibody association
  - Nerve conduction study shows conduction **block/focal** demyelination
- Treatment
  - IVIG, but NOT corticosteroids
    - Autoimmune sensory neuronopathy (ganglionopathy)
      1. Proximal and distal sensory loss
      2. Ataxia and pseudoathetosis
      3. Associated with GD1b antibodies

## VASCULITIC NEUROPATHY

Vasculitic Neuropathies present with multifocal weakness, sensory loss, or painful, burning paresthesias. These neuropathies result from transmural inflammation of the nerve, necrosis of epineural or perineural blood vessels, or deposition of immunoglobulin and membrane attack complex (MAC). Secondary vasculitides are caused by connective tissue diseases (eg, Sjögren), infection, malignancy, drug hypersensitivity, or cryoglobulins.

*Brachial Neuritis*

- Epidemiology: Male predominance (age 20-30 years old)
- Symptoms
  - Acute: Severe neuropathic pain in shoulder, arm, and/or hand that does not respond to NSAIDs
  - Days to weeks later: Weakness, muscle atrophy and sensory loss in affected limb with patchy nerve involvement
- Etiologies: Neuralgic amyotrophy, Parsonage-Turner syndrome
- Treatment: Complete recovery following physical therapy and analgesia (diclofenac or morphine acutely and gabapentin chronically), but can take 2 to 3 years

*Diabetic Lumbosacral Plexopathy (Diabetic Amyotrophy)*

- Symptoms
  - Severe, unilateral hip/thigh/low back pain with mild tingling/numbness which resolves
  - Weakness/atrophy which lasts for weeks, months, and occasionally permanent
  - Association with diabetes
- Diagnostics
  - CSF protein normal to mildly elevated
  - ESR can be elevated
- Treatment
  - Prednisone, but use with caution in diabetics

*Peripheral Neurosarcoidosis*

- Symptoms
  - Relapsing and remitting mononeuropathies, especially cranial nerves
- Diagnosis
  - CXR: Hilar adenopathy
  - ACE levels unhelpful
  - Noncaseating granulomas within and around peripheral nerves and associated blood vessels
- Treatment
  - Glucocorticoids
  - Immunosuppression (eg, methotrexate, azathioprine)
  - NSAIDs for symptom relief

*Stiff-Person Syndrome*

- Symptoms
  - Progressive rigidity and spasms of the trunk and limbs
  - Encephalomyelitis
  - Spasms worse with startle, emotions
  - 30% develop diabetes
- Laboratory
  - GAD antibodies (correlation with diabetes)
  - Anti-amphiphysin antibodies
  - CK elevation
- Treatment
  - Diazepam, gabapentin (GABAergic medications)
  - Baclofen
  - IVIG, plasma exchange, corticosteroids can occasionally help

## INFECTIOUS NEUROPATHIES

*Leprosy*

- Epidemiology: Common in Southeast Asia, South America, Africa, Texas, Hawaii, Florida. Armadillos are a natural reservoir.
  - Three disease types (lepromatous, tuberculoid, and borderline)
  - Transmitted via nasal droplets

- Diagnosis made on skin or nerve biopsy
- Treatment: Dapsone, rifampin

*Lyme*

- Epidemiology: Caused by *Borrelia burgdorferi* in the northeast and western Great Lakes areas. Infections usually occur from May to September
- Transmission: After tick attachment for 24 to 48 hours
- Symptoms
  - Stage 1: Erythema migrans, central pallor "bull's eye" rash (Fig. 9-1)
  - Stage 2: Dissemination, hematogenous spread, cranial neuropathies, cardiac complications
  - Stage 3: Chronic, distal symmetric polyneuropathy
- Treatment
  - Doxycycline or amoxicillin for erythema migrans and arthritis
  - Ceftriaxone for neurologic or cardiac Lyme

*HIV Neuropathy*

- Symptoms
  - Chronic and progressive distal sensory polyneuropathy: Severe ataxia
  - AIDP or CIDP
  - Polyradiculopathy
  - Multiple mononeuropathies secondary to vasculitic processes
- Treatment: Adequate control of HIV infection and avoidance of neuropathy-inducing HIV medications

*Human T-Lymphocytic Virus (HTLV-1)*

- Signs and symptoms
  - Tropical spastic paraparesis
  - Sensory polyneuropathy and/or myopathy
  - Can present with adult T-cell leukemia or lymphoma

*Cytomegalovirus (CMV)*

- Acute polyradiculopathy, especially lumbosacral

*Epstein-Barr Virus (EBV)*

- Associated with AIDP

**KEY FACT**

Congenital CMV infection CNS manifestations—microcephaly, ventriculomegaly, intracranial calcifications, sensorineural hearing loss

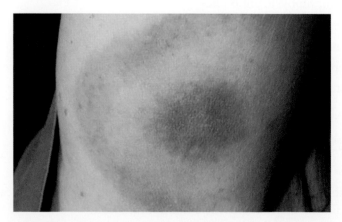

**FIGURE 9-1. Erythema migrans rash seen in Lyme disease.** https://www.cdc.gov/lyme/signs_symptoms/rashes.html

*Varicella Zoster Virus (VZV)*

- Etiology: Reactivation of latent dorsal root ganglia neurons
- Symptoms
  - Shingles/zoster
    - Vesicular rash and pain in dermatomal distribution
  - Postherpetic neuralgia
    - Sensory loss lasting over 1 month
  - Ramsay Hunt syndrome
    - Viral reactivation in facial nerve ganglion
    - Facial weakness with vesicular rash in external auditory canal
    - Hyperacusis, dizziness, hearing loss
    - Dysgeusia (abnormal taste)

*Hepatitis B and C*

- Hepatitis vasculitis: Mononeuritis multiplex
- HCV and type 3 cryoglobulinemia: Distal sensory polyneuropathy

*Diphtheria*

- Pathophysiology: Diphtheria toxin binds to Schwann cells in nerve roots and dorsal root ganglia
- Symptoms
  - Myalgias and fever
  - 50% of patients develop neuropathy: Bulbar weakness, autonomic dysfunction, blurred vision

## TOXIC NEUROPATHIES

*Chemotherapy*

- Taxanes: Paclitaxel, docetaxel
- Vinca alkaloids: Vincristine, vinblastine
- Platinum agents: Cisplatin; interferes with DNA repair

*Heavy Metals*

- **Arsenic**
  - Symptoms: Abdominal pain, nausea, vomiting, diarrhea
  - Signs: **Mees** lines in fingernails and toenails
  - Diagnostics: Pancytopenia and basophilic stippling of RBCs
  - Treatment: Chelation
    - Dimercaprol, succimer
- Lead
  - Signs: Radial neuropathy with wrist drop
  - Diagnostics: Microcytosis, hypochromia
  - Treatment: Chelation
    - Dimercaprol, succimer, EDTA
- Mercury
  - Signs: Encephalopathy, psychosis, ataxia
  - Diagnostics: Mercury levels in blood or urine

- Treatment: Chelation
  - Dimercaprol, succimer
- Thallium
  - Found in rat poison
  - Signs and symptoms
    - Alopecia, uremia, hepatic dysfunction
    - Mees lines in nails
  - Diagnostics: Thallium levels in blood or urine
  - Treatment: Prussian blue
- **Copper**
  - Pathophysiology: Wilson disease or ingestion of copper (eg, water through copper pipes)
  - Signs: **Kayser-Fleischer** rings
  - Symptoms: GI distress, melena, headache, dizziness, fatigue
  - Diagnostics: Increased serum copper or ceruloplasmin; increased copper excretion on urinalysis
  - Treatment: Penicillamine, trietine
- **Iron**
  - Pathophysiology: Recurrent blood transfusions, hemochromatosis
  - Signs: Hyperpigmentation of skin ("**bronze diabetes**"), cirrhosis, diabetes
  - Symptoms: Arthropathy, weakness, fatigue
  - Diagnostics: Anion gap metabolic acidosis, elevated liver enzymes (AST, ALT)
  - Treatment: Chelation
    - Deferoxamine, deferasirox, deferiprone
- Alcohol
  - Direct toxic effect and nutritional deficiency (B vitamins, folate)

## NUTRITIONAL NEUROPATHIES

*B1 Thiamine*

- Deficiency: Alcohol use disorder
- Symptoms: Beriberi
  - Symmetrical peripheral neuropathy and weakness (muscle wasting)
  - Dry (no CHF) vs wet (CHF, edema)

*B6 Pyridoxine*

- Symptoms: Seizures, peripheral neuropathy, and sideroblastic anemia (heme synthesis disruption)
- Deficiency: Associated with isoniazid and hydralazine use
- Toxicity: Excess supplementation

*B12 Cobalamin*

- Pathophysiology: B12 is a cofactor for DNA synthesis
- Deficiency: Diet (vegetarians), lack of intrinsic factor (gastrectomy, terminal ileum disease, pernicious anemia), nitrous oxide exposure

---

**WARDS TIP**

Administer thiamine before glucose/dextrose to prevent exacerbation of encephalopathy.

- Symptoms
  - Encephalopathy, subacute combined degeneration
  - Posterior columns: Decreased vibration and position
  - Corticospinal tracts: Hyperreflexia, weakness
- Diagnostics: Macrocytic anemia (can be masked with folate supplementation)
- Treatment: Intramuscular B12 replacement

### Vitamin E Deficiency

- Pathophysiology: Fat malabsorption and disorders of lipid metabolism
- Symptoms: Non-length-dependent sensory loss resulting in ataxia and gait instability

## IDIOPATHIC AND HEREDITARY NEUROPATHIES

### Amyotrophic Lateral Sclerosis (ALS)

- Pathophysiology: 10% familial; SOD1 mutation
- Subtypes: Primary muscular atrophy, progressive bulbar palsy, primary lateral sclerosis
- Symptoms
  - Slowly progressive asymmetric weakness → spreads to bulbar and respiratory weakness
  - Extraocular muscles and bowel/bladder spared
  - Lower Motor Neuron (LMN) dysfunction (eg, fasciculations, atrophy, cramps)
  - Upper Motor Neuron (UMN) dysfunction (eg, spasticity, slowness, hyperreflexia, clonus)
  - Pseudobulbar affect
- Diagnostics
  - EMG/NCS: Motor denervation/reinnervation without demyelination
  - CK mild-to-moderate elevation
- Treatment
  - Riluzole: Does not increase life expectancy. Possible GI side effects
  - Gastrostomy
  - Noninvasive ventilation with/without tracheostomy

### Spinal Muscular Atrophy (SMA)

- Subtypes
  - Type 1 (Werdnig-Hoffman)
    - Age of onset: Birth to 6 months
    - Floppy baby: Frog-leg posturing
    - Diminished deep tendon reflexes
    - Bulbar palsy or respiratory failure
  - Type 2
    - Age of onset: 6 to 18 months
    - Survival to second or third decade
    - Fine hand tremor and other musculoskeletal anomalies (eg, scoliosis)

- Type 3
  - Age of onset: 18 months to adulthood
  - Axial and respiratory weakness
  - Arthralgia and myalgia
  - can ambulate
- Pathophysiology: Autosomal recessive mutation in SMN gene on chromosome 5q
- Treatment: Supportive

*Charcot-Marie-Tooth Disease (Hereditary Motor Sensory Neuropathy)*

- Most common type of hereditary neuropathy, resulting from a mutation in the CMT1 gene
- Symptoms
  - Distal weakness
  - Steppage gait (foot drop)
  - Pes cavus (high arched feet; Fig. 9-2)
- Diagnostics
  - EMG/NCS: Motor and sensory nerve conduction affected
  - Nerve biopsy: "Onion bulb" Schwann cells
  - Various mutations including PMP-22 duplication

## Radiculopathies and Plexopathies

Radiculopathies are caused by spinal cord nerve root compression and plexopathies involve disorders of either the brachial or lumbosacral plexi (Tables 9-1 and 9-2).

- Cervical radiculopathies
  - Symptoms: Pain, hypesthesia or paresthesia, weakness, reduced upper extremity reflexes
  - Cause: Ligament hypertrophy, disk protrusion
  - Diagnosis
    - Spurling sign: Limb pain/paresthesia is reproduced with neck extension and rotation toward the symptomatic side
    - EMG/NCS: Differentiates radiculopathy from plexopathy
    - MRI or CT myelogram
  - Treatment: Most are self-limiting or effectively treated with physical therapy and exercise. Further treatment options include:
    - Epidural steroid injections
    - Surgical decompression for weakness, worsening sensory loss, and severe pain

## TABLE 9-1. Upper Extremity Nerves and Related Radiculopathies

| Nerve | Causes of Injury | Presentation |
|---|---|---|
| Axillary (C5-C6) | Fractured surgical neck of humerus; anterior dislocation of humerus | Flattened deltoid<br>Loss of arm abduction at shoulder (>15°)<br>Loss of sensation over deltoid muscle and lateral arm |
| Musculocutaneous (C5-C7) | Upper trunk compression | Loss of forearm flexion and supination<br>Loss of sensation over lateral forearm |
| Radial (C5-T1) | Midshaft fracture of humerus; compression of axilla, eg, due to crutches or sleeping with arm over chair ("Saturday night palsy") | Wrist drop: loss of elbow, wrist, and finger extension<br>↓ Grip strength (wrist extension necessary for maximal action of flexors)<br>Loss of sensation over posterior arm/forearm and dorsal hand |
| Median (C5-T1) | Supracondylar fracture of humerus (proximal lesion); carpal tunnel syndrome and wrist laceration (distal lesion) | "Ape hand" and "Pope's blessing"<br>Loss of wrist flexion, flexion of lateral fingers, thumb opposition, lumbricals of 2nd and 3rd digits<br>Loss of sensation over thenar eminence and dorsal and palmar aspects of lateral 3½ fingers with proximal lesion |
| Ulnar (C8-T1) | Fracture of medial epicondyle of humerus "funny bone" (proximal lesion); fractured hook of hamate (distal lesion) from fall on outstretched hand | "Ulnar claw" on digit extension<br>Radial deviation of wrist upon flexion (proximal lesion)<br>Loss of wrist flexion, flexion of medial fingers, abduction and adduction of fingers (interossei), actions of medial 2 lumbrical muscles<br>Loss of sensation over medial 1½ fingers including hypothenar eminence |
| Recurrent branch of median nerve (C5-T1) | Superficial laceration of palm | "Ape hand"<br>Loss of thenar muscle group: opposition, abduction, and flexion of thumb<br>No loss of sensation |

Reproduced with permission from Bhushan V., Le T. First Aid for the USMLE Step 1 2017. New York: McGraw Hill; 2017.

## TABLE 9-2. Brachial Plexopathies and Upper Limb Focal Neuropathies

| Condition | Injury | Causes | Muscle Deficit | Functional Deficit | Presentation |
|---|---|---|---|---|---|
| **Erb palsy** ("waiter's tip") | Traction or tear of **upper** ("Erb-er") trunk: C5-C6 roots | Infants—lateral traction on neck during delivery Adults—trauma | Deltoid, supraspinatus Infraspinatus Biceps brachii | Abduction (arm hangs by side)<br>Lateral rotation (arm medially rotated)<br>Flexion, supination (arm extended and pronated) | |
| **Klumpke palsy** | Traction or tear of **lower** trunk: C8-T1 root | Infants—upward force on arm during delivery Adults—trauma (eg, grabbing a tree branch to break a fall) | Intrinsic hand muscles: lumbricals, interossei, thenar, hypothenar | Total claw hand: lumbricals normally flex MCP joints and extend DIP and PIP joints | |
| Thoracic outlet syndrome | Compression of **lower** trunk and subclavian vessels | Cervical rib (arrows in A), Pancoast tumor | Same as Klumpke palsy | Atrophy of intrinsic hand muscles; ischemia, pain, and edema due to vascular compression | |
| Winged scapula | Lesion of long thoracic nerve | Axillary node dissection after mastectomy, stab wounds | Serratus anterior | Inability to anchor scapula to thoracic cage → cannot abduct arm above horizontal position | |

Reproduced with permission from Bhushan V., Le T. First Aid for the USMLE Step 1 2017. New York: McGraw Hill; 2017.

■ Lumbosacral plexopathies

- Symptoms: Weakness and sensory loss from more than one root or nerve territory
- Causes: Diabetic amyotrophy, vasculitis, infectious (zoster, Lyme disease), trauma/compressive (ie, surgery, obstetric, aortic/iliac aneurysm)

■ Lumbosacral radiculopathies

- Symptoms: Pain or paresthesia, reduced reflexes, and muscle weakness
- Causes: Disc herniation, ligament hypertrophy, osteophytes, synovial cysts, tumor, infectious masses
  – Individual nerve pathologies are detailed in Table 9-3
- Treatment: Physical therapy, epidural steroids, or decompressive surgery when weakness is severe/worsening

Nerves and arteries are frequently named together by the bones/regions with which they are associated. The exceptions to this naming convention are listed in Table 9-4.

**TABLE 9-3. Lower Extremity Nerves and Associated Radiculopathies**

| Nerve | Innervation | Cause of Injury | Presentation/Comments |
|---|---|---|---|
| Iliohypogastric (T12-L1) | Sensory—suprapubic region Motor—transversus abdominis and internal oblique | Abdominal surgery | Burning or tingling pain in surgical incision site radiating to inguinal and suprapubic region |
| Genitofemoral nerve (L1-L2) | Sensory—scrotum/labia majora, medial thigh Motor—cremaster | Laparoscopic surgery | ↓ Anterior thigh sensation beneath inguinal ligament; absent cremasteric reflex |
| Lateral femoral cutaneous (L2-L3) | Sensory—anterior and lateral thigh | Tight clothing, obesity, pregnancy | ↓ Thigh sensation (anterior and lateral) |
| Obturator (L2-L4) | Sensory—medial thigh Motor—obturator externus, adductor longus, adductor brevis, gracilis, pectineus, adductor magnus | Pelvic surgery | ↓ Thigh sensation (medial) and adduction |
| Femoral (L2-L4) | Sensory—anterior thigh, medial leg Motor—quadriceps, iliopsoas, pectineus, sartorius | Pelvic fracture | ↓ Thigh flexion and leg extension |
| Sciatic (L4-S3) | Sensory—posterior thigh Motor—semitendinosus, semimembranosus, biceps femoris, adductor magnus | Herniated disc | Splits into common peroneal and tibial nerves |
| Common peroneal (L4-S2) | Sensory—dorsum of foot Motor—biceps femoris, tibialis anterior, extensor muscles of foot | Trauma or compression of lateral aspect of leg, fibular neck fracture | PED = Peroneal Everts and Dorsiflexes; if injured, foot dropPED Loss of sensation on dorsum of foot Foot drop—inverted and plantarflexed at rest, loss of eversion and dorsiflexion; "steppage gait" |
| Tibial (L4-S3) | Sensory—sole of foot Motor—triceps surae, plantaris, popliteus, flexor muscles of foot | Knee trauma, Baker cyst (proximal lesion); tarsal tunnel syndrome (distal lesion) | TIP = Tibial Inverts and Plantarflexes; if injured, can't stand on TIPtoes Inability to curl toes and loss of sensation on sole; in proximal lesions, foot everted at rest with loss of inversion and plantarflexion |

| | | | |
|---|---|---|---|
| Superior gluteal (L4-S1)<br><br>Normal   Trendelenburg sign<br> | Motor—gluteus medius, gluteus minimus, tensor fascia latae | Iatrogenic injury during intramuscular injection to upper medial gluteal region | Trendelenburg sign/gait—pelvis tilts because weight-bearing leg cannot maintain alignment of pelvis through hip abduction<br>Lesion is contralateral to the side of the hip that drops, ipsilateral to extremity on which the patient stands<br>Choose superolateral quadrant (ideally the anterolateral region) as intramuscular injection site to avoid nerve injury |
| Inferior gluteal (L5-S2) | Motor—gluteus maximus | Posterior hip dislocation | Difficulty climbing stairs, rising from seated position; loss of hip extension |
| Pudendal (S2-S4) | Sensory—perineum<br>Motor—external urethral and anal sphincters | Stretch injury during childbirth | ↓ Sensation in perineum and genital area; can cause fecal or urinary incontinence<br>Can be blocked with local anesthetic during childbirth using ischial spine as a landmark for injection |

Reproduced with permission from Bhushan V., Le T. First Aid for the USMLE Step 1 2017. New York: McGraw Hill; 2017.

### TABLE 9-4. Neurovascular Pairing

| Location | Nerve | Artery |
|---|---|---|
| Axilla/lateral thorax | Long thoracic | Lateral thoracic |
| Surgical neck of humerus | Axillary | Posterior circumflex |
| Midshaft of humerus | Radial | Deep brachial |
| Distal humerus/cubital fossa | Median | Brachial |
| Popliteal fossa | Tibial | Popliteal |
| Posterior to medial malleolus | Tibial | Posterior tibial |

Reproduced with permission from Bhushan V., Le T. First Aid for the USMLE Step 1 2017. New York: McGraw Hill; 2017.

## ENDOCRINOPATHIES

*Diabetic Neuropathies*

- Distal symmetric sensory polyneuropathy
- Cranial neuropathies and mononeuropathies
  - Ophthalmoparesis and ptosis
  - Compressive neuropathies such as carpal tunnel, peroneal neuropathy
- Autonomic neuropathy
  - Constipation, orthostatic changes, dry eyes/mouth, sexual dysfunction
- Proximal neuropathies
  - Brachial neuritis

*Hypothyroidism*

- Carpel tunnel syndrome
- Distal symmetric sensory polyneuropathy

## SYSTEMIC DISEASES

*Uremic Neuropathy*

- Distal symmetric polyneuropathy
- Caused by urea and other waste product accumulation

**KEY FACT**

With median nerve compression can often see Tinel's sign (positive if percussion of a nerve reproduces symptoms). Also, Phalen's sign (wrists held in flexed posture for 60 seconds. Positive if symptoms reproduced/worsen).

**KEY FACT**

In foot drop, weakness of ankle inversion distinguishes peroneal neuropathy from L5 radiculopathy or sciatic neuropathy. Tibialis posterior (L5-S1, sciatic nerve, tibial nerve) is not weak in peroneal neuropathy.

*Malabsorption Syndromes*

■ Distal symmetric sensory polyneuropathy

■ Vitamin deficiency: B12, E, copper

*Critical Illness*

■ Severe neuropathy or myopathy in the setting of multiple organ failure, failing to wean from ventilator, prolonged high-dose steroid use

## MALIGNANCIES

Malignancies lead to neuropathies via direct invasion, autoimmunity or paraneoplastic syndromes, paraprotein-related etiologies, or secondary to chemotherapy or radiation. The following pathologies are all paraproteinemias.

*Multiple Myeloma*

■ Multiple myeloma is cancer that affects plasma cells

■ Caused by a monoclonal gammopathy leading to distal axonal sensory and motor damage

 • Produces large amounts of IgG and IgA

■ Symptoms: Fatigue, bone pain, hypercalcemia, anemia

■ POEMS variant

 • Polyneuropathy (symmetric)

 • Organomegaly (hepatosplenomegaly, ascites, papilledema)

 • Endocrinopathy (hypothyroidism, gynecomastia, testicular atrophy, amenorrhea)

 • Monoclonal gammopathy

 • Skin changes (hyperpigmentation, hypertrichosis, edema, clubbing)

 • Associated with elevated VEGF (vascular endothelial growth factor), reduced erythropoietin, other malignancies

*Monoclonal Gammopathy of Unknown Significance (MGUS)*

■ Neuropathy caused by distal demyelination

■ Symptoms: Ataxia

*Waldenstrom Gammaglobulinemia*

■ Neuropathy caused by accumulation of IgM

■ Symptoms: Anemia, fatigue, lymphoplasmacytoid cells

*Amyloidosis*

■ AA protein accumulation resulting in a connective tissue disease

■ Symptoms: Distal paresthesia, autonomic symptoms, compressive neuropathies

■ FAP: Familial transthyretin, apolipoprotein A-1

## DISORDERS OF THE NEUROMUSCULAR JUNCTION

*Myasthenia Gravis (Autoimmune)*

■ Can have Co-occurrence with other autoimmune disorders (ie, hyperthyroidism)

■ Symptoms

 • Muscle fatigability with repeated actions

 • Dysphagia, diplopia, ptosis, dyspnea, neck extensor weakness

- Signs
  - Cogan's lid twitch sign - elicited by asking the patient to gaze downward for 10–15 seconds and then returning to primary gaze. Cogan's sign is present when the affected lid briefly "twitches" upward on returning to primary gaze.
- Types
  - Generalized: Affecting limbs, facial muscles and even respiratory muscles
  - Ocular: Ptosis and ophthalmoparesis only
  - Neonatal: Placental transfer of maternal IgG against AChR; resolves in weeks and responsive to cholinesterase inhibitors
- Pathophysiology
  - IgG antibodies against nicotinic acetylcholine receptor → reduces number of receptors
- Diagnosis
  - Anti-AChR antibodies in blood
  - Seronegative patients may have MuSK antibodies (muscle-specific tyrosine kinase)
  - CT chest: Thymoma
  - EMG/NCS: Decrement in amplitude with repetitive stimulation
  - Edrophonium (Tensilon) test: Cholinesterase inhibitor administration
- Treatment
  - Cholinesterase inhibitors
    - Pyridostigmine: Increases availability of Ach at neuromuscular junction
  - Immunosuppression/Immunomodulation
    - Prednisone
    - Azathioprine: Hepatotoxicity, bone marrow suppression, pancreatitis
    - Cyclosporine A: Nephrotoxicity, contraindicated in pregnancy
    - Mycophenolate
    - Plasma exchange
    - IVIG
  - Thymectomy

## Lambert-Eaton Myasthenic Syndrome (LEMS; Autoimmune)

- Epidemiology: Affects >40 years old
- Symptoms
  - Weakness and fatigability in proximal muscles
  - Improves with repeated action
  - Autonomic symptoms
- Pathophysiology
  - Antibodies to voltage-gated calcium channels which interfere with binding/release of vesicles containing Ach
  - Paraneoplastic with small cell lung cancer correlation

## Botulism

- Pathophysiology: Caused by *Clostridium botulinum* toxin
  - Foodborne: Develops over 12 to 36 hours (Canned foods)

- Wound: Develops over days to weeks
- Infantile: Poor feeding, hypotonia (Can occur after consuming honey)
- Symptoms
  - Diarrhea, nausea, vomiting, diplopia, dysarthria, ptosis
  - Generalized weakness particularly bulbar muscles
- Treatment: Supportive with antitoxin only helpful within 24 hours after symptom onset

### Tick Paralysis

- Pathophysiology: Blockage of NMJ transmission
  - Caused by wood and dog ticks
- Symptoms: Rapidly ascending weakness
- Treat with tick removal and supportive care

### Presynaptic Toxins

- Sodium channels
  - Tetrodotoxin: Japanese pufferfish
  - Saxitoxin: Shellfish
  - Ciguatoxin: Reef fish; abdominal pain, oral paresthesias, altered temperature
- Potassium channels
  - Aminopyridines
  - Dendrotoxin (black and green mamba)
- Calcium channels
  - Verapamil, diltiazem: Worsen myasthenia
- Antibiotics: Aminoglycosides can alter NMJ transmission

### Synaptic Toxins (Anticholinesterases)

- Organophosphates and insecticides
- Signs and symptoms
  - Muscle twitching, pinpoint pupils, flaccid paralysis
  - Nausea, vomiting, sweating, abdominal cramps, bradycardia, salivation
- Treatment: Atropine, pralidoxime

### Postsynaptic Toxins

- Curare
- Aminoglycosides, tetracyclines, procainamide, penicillamine
- α-Bungarotoxin

### Stiff-Person Syndrome

- Symptoms
  - Progressive rigidity and spasms of the trunk and limbs, with or without encephalomyelitis
  - Spasms worsened by stimulation, startle, emotions (external or internal stimuli)
  - Other autoimmune conditions such as diabetes DM Type 1, myasthenia gravis, thyroiditis, SLE, and RA
- Laboratory
  - Anti-glutamic acid decarboxylase (GAD) antibodies in 60%

- Some have anti-amphiphysin antibodies
- Elevated creatine kinase
- Pathophysiology
  - GAD synthesizes gamma-aminobutyric acid (GABA) from glutamic acid; reduced inhibition of upper motor neurons → hyperactivity
  - GAD present in pancreatic islet cells → diabetes
  - Spontaneous or paraneoplastic (especially lymphoma, small cell lung cancer, breast cancer)
- Treatment
  - GABAergic medications (eg, diazepam, gabapentin)
  - Baclofen (PO or intrathecal)
  - Immunomodulation (eg, IVIG, plasma exchange, corticosteroids) can help

## AUTOIMMUNE AND INFLAMMATORY MYOPATHIES

### Polymyositis/Dermatomyositis

- Symptoms
  - Proximal > distal weakness (shoulder, hip girdle weakness)
  - Dysphagia
  - Skin changes: Heliotrope rash, shawl sign, Gottron papules (papular rash over knuckles)
  - Interstitial lung disease
- Diagnostics
  - CK moderately elevated
  - EMG myopathic
  - Jo-1 antibody
  - Pulmonary function tests: Restrictive lung disease
- Pathophysiology
  - Associated with malignancy
  - Associated with SLE, Sjögrens, rheumatoid arthritis
  - Polymyositis
    - Endomysial CD8+ T cells
  - Dermatomyositis
    - Perifascicular atrophy, perivascular inflammation
- Treatment
  - Immunomodulation: Corticosteroids, azathioprine, methotrexate, IVIG, plasma exchange, mycophenolate, rituximab

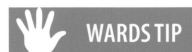 **WARDS TIP**

Paraneoplastic dermatosis may present as an erythematous rash distributed in a "shawl" pattern over the neck, upper back, chest and shoulders.

### Inclusion Body Myositis

- Epidemiology: Male predominance
- Symptoms
  - Asymmetric proximal > distal weakness and atrophy
  - Finger flexors, wrist flexors, and quadriceps
  - Dysphagia
- Diagnostics
  - CK mild-to-moderate elevation

- Histopathology: Inclusion bodies (rimmed vacuoles), mononuclear invasion of non-necrotic fibers, intracellular amyloid deposits
- Treatment: Does not respond to immune therapies

## HEREDITARY MYOPATHIES

*Duchenne Muscular Dystrophy*

- Epidemiology: Age 2 to 6
- Pathophysiology: Spontaneous loss of function mutation in dystrophin gene
- Signs and symptoms
  - Waddling gait with slow running due to proximal weakness
  - Gower's sign: Patient has to use their hands and arms to "walk" up their own body from a squatting position due to lack of hip and thigh muscle strength
  - Calf pseudohypertrophy: Calf appears muscular but in fact is enlarged due to fibrosis
  - Death from respiratory or cardiac failure (dilated cardiomyopathy)
- Diagnostics
  - CK 50-100× upper limit of normal
  - DNA testing with dystrophin gene deletion
  - Pathology shows necrotic/regenerating muscle fibers and increased connective tissue
- Treatment: Supportive, corticosteroids

*Becker Muscular Dystrophy*

- Pathophysiology: Truncation or partial loss of dystrophin
- Signs and symptoms
  - Phenotype and histopathology similar to Duchenne but less severe
  - Walking until age 15, but 40% cannot walk by age 30

*Myotonic Dystrophy*

- Pathophysiology
  - Autosomal dominant
  - Type 1: CTG repeat expansion in DMPK gene
  - Type 2: CCTG repeat expansion in DMPK gene
- Signs and symptoms
  - Progressive distal → proximal weakness
  - Myotonia (delayed muscle relaxation after forced contraction) that improves with repetition (classically difficulty releasing handshake)
  - Intellectual disability, cataracts, cardiomyopathy, male-pattern baldness, sleep apnea
- Diagnostics
  - EMG: Myotonic discharges
- Treatment
  - Mexiletine or phenytoin for myotonia
  - Management of cardiomyopathy

# GLYCOGEN STORAGE DISEASES

*Type II (Pompe Disease)*

- Pathophysiology: Defect in alpha-1,4-glucosidase which leads to glycogen accumulation
- Signs and symptoms
  - Infants: Generalized weakness/hypotonia, cardiomegaly, hepatomegaly, macroglossia, respiratory failure
  - Juvenile: Gower sign, waddling gait
  - Adults: Respiratory failure
- Diagnostics
  - Muscle biopsy shows glycogen-filled PAS+ subsarcolemmal vacuoles
- Treatment: IV recombinant alpha-glucosidase

*Type V (McArdle Disease)*

- Most common glycolytic/glycogenolytic disorder
- Pathophysiology: Autosomal recessive inheritance of a deficiency of myophosphorylase leads to glycogen accumulation within the muscle
- Signs and symptoms
  - Exercise intolerance, muscle pain, cramping
  - Second-wind phenomenon: Initial myalgias and cramping improve as blood glucose is activated
  - Myoglobinuria
- Treatment: Oral sucrose loading before exercise can improve tolerance

# LIPID AND FREE FATTY ACID METABOLISM DISEASES

*CPT II Deficiency*

- Pathophysiology: Autosomal recessive CPT II deficiency results in impaired acylcarnitine transport at the inner mitochondrial membrane
- Signs and symptoms
  - Myalgia provoked by prolonged/intense exercise, illness, fasting
- Treatment: Treat with high-protein and low-fat diet and avoid prolonged exertion/fasting

*Carnitine Transporter Deficiency*

- Pathophysiology: Mutation in carnitine transporter protein OCTN2 resulting in carnitine deficiency
- Signs and symptoms: Vomiting, confusion, hepatic dysfunction

# CHANNELOPATHIES

*Malignant Hyperthermia*

- Pathophysiology
  - Mutations in ryanodine receptor RyR1
  - Caused by depolarizing NMJ blockers and inhaled anesthetics
- Signs and symptoms
  - Severe muscle rigidity, myoglobinuria
  - High fever, tachycardia, arrhythmias
- Treatment: Dantrolene and aggressive cooling

**Case 1:** A 57-year-old man presents to the physician because of a 2-month history of intermittent drooping of his left eyelid each evening and occasional difficulty chewing and swallowing. He also reports two episodes of double vision while reading that occurred in the evening and resolved by the following morning. Examination shows no abnormalities except for slight ptosis on the left. Which of the following is the most likely diagnosis?

A. Acute intermittent porphyria
B. Myasthenia gravis
C. Complex partial seizures
D. Guillain-Barre syndrome
E. Brain stem glioma

The correct answer is B. The combination of ptosis, intermittent double vision, and trouble with chewing and swallowing is concerning for myasthenia gravis.

**Case 2:** A 53-year-old man has had a 3-week history of increasing neck pain when he turns his head to the left. He also has had a pins-and-needles sensation starting in the neck and radiating down the left arm into the thumb. Neurologic examination shows limitation of motion on turning the neck to the left. There is 4+/5 weakness of the left biceps and decreased pinprick over the left thumb. Deep tendon reflexes are 1+ in the left biceps and brachioradialis; all others are 2+. Which of the following is the most likely diagnosis?

A. Carpal tunnel syndrome
B. Thoracic outlet syndrome
C. Multiple sclerosis
D. Cervical root compression
E. Radial nerve compression

The correct answer is D. Cervical root compression since the patient has radicular pain in the distribution of a cervical root on the left.

**Case 3:** A 35-year-old administrative assistant has had severe episodic pain in her right thumb and right second and third digits for 3 months. The pain started as intermittent pins and needles but now frequently awakens her from sleep. She has decreased sensation over the palmar surface of the thumb and index finger of the right hand and atrophy of the thenar muscle mass. By tapping on the wrist, the physician can elicit pins-and-needles sensation in her hand. Compression of which of the following nerves is the most likely cause?

A. Median
B. Musculocutaneous
C. Posterior interosseous
D. Radial
E. Ulnar

The correct answer is A. The patient is suffering from carpal tunnel syndrome and has compression of the median nerve. Tinel's test helps confirm the diagnosis as does the distribution of her paresthesia.

# CHAPTER 10

# EPILEPSY AND
# SEIZURE DISORDERS

In this chapter, we will review seizures, which are an abnormality of cerebral electrical activity.

A combination of tools and clinical signs are used to categorize this pathology including electroencephalograms (EEGs) which sample cerebral electrical activity with an array of electrodes placed onto the scalp. There are a multitude of antiseizure medications that can be tailored by onset time, efficacy, and side-effect profile. Patients with seizures refractory to multiple medications may be eligible for surgical interventions to help reduce the frequency and intensity of their seizures.

## Seizure Disorders

**Seizure:** Abnormal electrical discharges among a group of neurons that persists long enough to interrupt normal functioning of that region of the brain.

**Epilepsy:** Disorder defined by a tendency toward multiple unprovoked seizures. Approximately 1% of the US population and 65 million people worldwide suffer from epilepsy. There is a bimodal presentation of the disease appearing most often in childhood (influenced by genetic abnormalities) and second most often in the elderly (often related to cerebral injuries including stroke).

Depending on the area of involvement, there may be associated contractions of groups of muscles, changes in sensation, or alterations in consciousness during an episode. These signs are typically stereotyped at each episode and can help approximate seizure focus in the brain and progression throughout the brain.

### FOCAL SEIZURE

- Seizures originating in one hemisphere, even if from multiple onset zones, and spreading only to regions within this hemisphere.
  - Signs and symptoms (brain region dependent): Sensation change early in focal seizures is common and is called an aura.
    - Typically, these include metallic taste, nausea, stomach upswelling sensation, déjà vu, vision changes, fear, panic, or euphoria. The stereotyped presentation favors a focal electrographic seizure.
  - May have perfectly intact awareness (simple) or impaired awareness at any point during the event (complex).

### SECONDARILY GENERALIZED SEIZURE

- Onset in one hemisphere, ideally as detected on EEG or with clear focal motor movement, with electrical spread to networks within both hemispheres.
- Typically causes loss of awareness and bilateral motor movements.

### GENERALIZED SEIZURE

- Activation of a network of abnormal epileptogenic that involves both hemispheres simultaneously. Starts with loss of awareness.

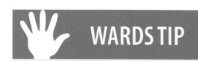

**WARDS TIP**

Complex focal seizure presents with automatisms (lip smacking, hand rubbing, leg bicycling, eye fluttering, etc.) and most often have loss of awareness/impaired consciousness.

## MYOCLONIC SEIZURE

- Contraction of either a single or group of muscles that coincides with abnormal electrographic discharge. Nonrhythmic and irregular jerks.
  - Subcortical myoclonic event: electrographic discharge(s) originating near or below the level of the deeper gray nuclei most commonly with uninhibited spinal circuits after diffuse cortical injury or direct trauma.

## TONIC-CLONIC SEIZURE (GRAND MAL)

- Tonic Phase: Excessive activation from the group of neurons causes a forced extension of the limb(s).
  - Typically occurs first, before the clonic phase.
  - Compared to an atonic (astatic) seizure which includes a sudden loss of tone ("drop attack") due to a variation of how the motor network is interrupted.
  - Characteristic rotated eyes, tongue biting, apnea, tonic cry (moan).
- Clonic Phase: Rhythmic jerking of the limb(s) that typically appears later coinciding with periodic larger amplitude discharges. These larger discharges have longer neuronal refractory periods that allows the muscle to relax in between contractions.

## SUBCLINICAL SEIZURE

- Meets criteria for electrographic seizure but without an associated detectable motor or reported sensory change.
- Factors including the patient's condition (under sedation or paralysis), region of affected brain (if away from motor and sensory pathways), or temporal relationship to recent larger seizures are typical scenarios for the occurrence of subclinical seizures.

## STATUS EPILEPTICUS

A life-threatening condition in which the brain is in a state of persistent seizure. Definitions vary, but traditionally it is defined as one continuous unremitting seizure lasting longer than **30 minutes**, or recurrent seizures without regaining consciousness between seizures for >30 minutes. See Fig. 10-1.

- Most seizures last less than 2 to 3 minutes. If a seizure lasts >5 minutes, begin treatment for status epilepticus.
- Approximately 10% of people with epilepsy will go into status epilepticus at some point in their life.
- Most common in young children and the elderly.
- Antiepileptic drugs (AEDs) with IV formulation are phenytoin, valproate, phenobarbital, levetiracetam, and lacosamide.
- Status Epilepticus may be convulsive or non-convulsive.

**KEY FACT**

Approximately 80% of prolonged seizures are stopped with a 'combination of IV benzodiazepines and a first line anti-seizure medication'.

## EPILEPSIA PARTIALIS CONTINUA (EPC)

- EPC is a variant of simple focal motor status epilepticus in which frequent repetitive muscle jerks, usually arrhythmic, continue for long periods of time.
- EPC can happen every few seconds or minutes and can continue for days, weeks or even years.
- EPC seizures are most common in the hands and face (focal).

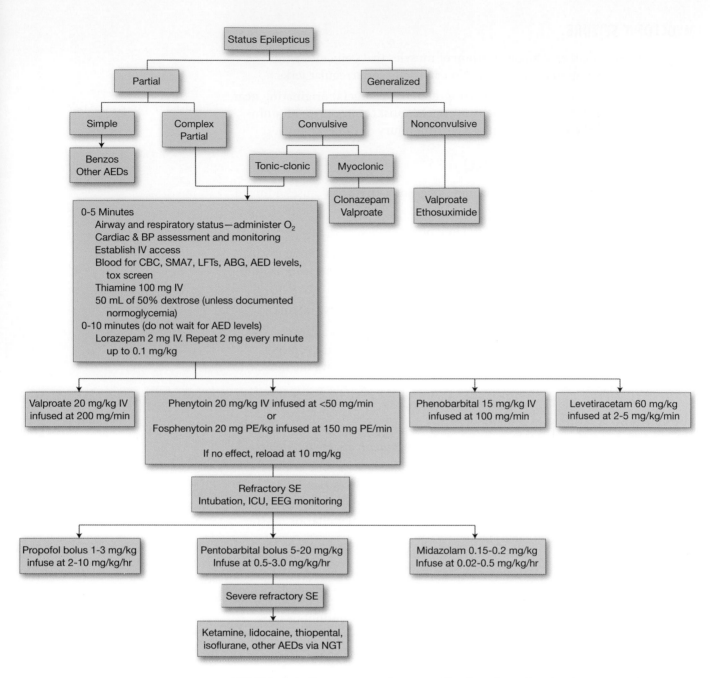

**FIGURE 10-1. Management of status epilepticus.** Reproduced with permission from Rafii M. et al. *First Aid for the Neurology Boards, 2nd ed.* New York: McGraw Hill; 2015.

## SUDDEN UNEXPECTED DEATH IN EPILEPSY (SUDEP)

■ Fatal complication of epilepsy occurring due to cardiopulmonary failure from ongoing seizure activity.

## PSYCHOGENIC NONEPILEPTIC SEIZURES (PNES)

■ Physical signs that mimic electrographic seizure driven by psychological stress without changes in brain electrical activity.

■ There is a small overlap (10%-20%) of patients with epilepsy who will also demonstrate some psychogenic episodes.

- Treated with psychological therapy and antidepressant or anxiolytic medications rather than antiseizure medications.
- PNES are also called pseudoseizures or psychogenic seizures and are a form of conversion disorder.

## FEBRILE SEIZURES

- Seizures associated with fever in children 6 months to 5 years of age without intracranial infection; average age 18 to 22 months; boys > girls.
- Approximately 1 in 25 children have febrile seizure and one-third will have a recurrence.
- Usually occurs the first day of a fever, sometimes before a fever is recognized.
- Seizures can be of any type—usually tonic-clonic or tonic.
- Complex if seizure lasts >15 minutes, more than one seizure in 24 hours, or focal features.
- EEG is generally not useful; epileptiform activity is not predictive of eventual development of epilepsy.
- ↑ risk of developing epilepsy (3% by age 7 vs 0.5% in the general population).

**Management:**

- Identify underlying illness and do lumbar puncture if there is clinical concern about meningitis.
- No neuroimaging is necessary unless the physical exam points to possible structural lesion.
- No treatment is necessary except lowering the fever; for children who have frequent or prolonged febrile seizures, oral or rectal diazepam during fevers can be used.

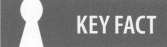

**KEY FACT**

PNES differentiators—most seizures in front of others and not in sleep.

## Principles of EEG

Electroencephalography (EEG): Electrodes placed on the scalp that can detect cerebral electrical activity.

- Normal electrographic background: on EEG, the result of the complex interplay of different brain regions generates countable shifts of electrical charge at the neuronal level.
  - These shifts are measured in terms of frequencies (Hz) ranging from 0 to >100 Hz.
  - Although multiple frequency ranges may overlap one another, there are expected ranges based on the patient's age, arousal state, and influence by external factors like medications.
- Interictal (between seizures): The EEG pattern between electrographic seizures.
  - If intermittent abnormal discharges are detected, depending on the pattern, these may convey an area of epileptogenic potential.
- EEG waves are named based on their frequency range using Greek numerals.
  - Beta Waves (frequency range from 14 Hz to about 30 Hz)
  - Alpha Waves (frequency range from 8.5 Hz to 13 Hz)
  - Theta Waves (frequency range from 4 Hz to 8.5 Hz)
  - Delta Waves (frequency range up to 3 Hz)

# Epilepsy Syndromes

There are several childhood epilepsy syndromes that are the result of genetic alterations to these ion channels which are diagnosed by their abnormal electrical signature and clinical presentation:

- Neonatal
  - **Benign fifth day fits**
    - Focal motor seizures between day 2 and 7 of life.
    - There is an autosomal-dominant version of this that affects the potassium ion channels called benign familial neonatal epilepsy (BFNE).
    - This spectrum can be treated with phenobarbital but usually remits within 1 to 2 days.
- Infancy (6 months to 2 years)
  - **Febrile seizure (simple vs complex)**
    - Ages 6 months to 5 years: typically generalized seizure associated with fever.
    - Occurs in 1 in 75 children and one-third of these will have a recurrence; 3% chance of developing epilepsy.
    - Complex febrile seizure: if the seizure lasts >15 minutes or more than one seizure in 24 hours or clear focal features.
    - MRI and EEG for complex seizures; not for simple seizure.
  - **Benign infantile myoclonic epilepsy**
    - 1 to 2 years of life
    - Brief recurrent generalized jerking (myoclonic) seizures treated with valproate.
  - **Dravet syndrome**
    - 1 to 2 years of life: severe, refractory frequent myoclonic seizures with impact on neurodevelopment.
    - SCN1A gene mutation (alpha subunit of voltage-gated sodium channel).
    - Treat with valproate then clobazam.
  - **West syndrome**
    - Those at risk: tuberous sclerosis patients, inborn errors of metabolism, neonatal brain injury.
    - Clinical criteria:
      - Infantile spasms ("jack-knifing" of arms and trunk) are first clinical symptom.
      - EEG shows chaotic high-amplitude background activity known as hypsarrhythmia (show example).
      - Child eventually demonstrates mental regression.
    - Treated with ACTH (adrenocortropic hormone), vigabatrin, and/or focal resective surgery if focal lesion found.
- Childhood (1- to 6-year-old)
  - **BECTS (Benign epilepsy with centrotemporal spikes/Rolandic epilepsy)**
    - 3 to 16 years of life.
    - Most common focal epilepsy of childhood that usually resolves by late teen years without neurocognitive impact.

- Nocturnal seizures with choking sounds and salivation are common.
- Treated with carbamazepine.
- **Childhood Absence Epilepsy (CAE)**
  - Age 2 through 13 years old: Behavioral arrest, eye fluttering, automatisms multiple times per day.
  - EEG shows bilaterally synchronous and symmetrical 3-Hz spike-and-wave discharges that start and end abruptly. If the seizures appear later in age, 10 to 17 years old, these seizures can be classified as juvenile absence epilepsy.
  - Treated with ethosuximide and valproic acid.
- **Lennox-Gastaut**
  - Age 1 to 10 years: Multiple seizure types, intellectual disability.
  - Slow spike-wave activity on EEG (1- to 2-Hz generalized discharges).
  - Usually refractory to multiple medications.
- **Rasmussen's Encephalitis**
  - Age 6 to 10 years: Uncontrollable focal seizures.
  - EPC is common where child will have near continuous stream of focal motor seizures meeting criteria for status epilepticus.
  - IVIG may be used but hemispherectomy is the most common treatment.
- Adolescence
  - Juvenile Absence Epilepsy (JAE)
    - Present predominantly with severe, noticeable absence seizures with or without a mild myoclonic component.
  - Juvenile Myoclonic Epilepsy (JME)
    - Present predominantly with myoclonic jerks upon waking from sleep, with or without a mild absence component.
- Other causes of seizure disorder
  - Alcohol withdrawal
    - Timing (24 to 48 hours after last drink)
    - Delirium Tremens
    - Treatment: thiamine before glucose, fast-acting benzodiazepine
  - **Posterior reversible encephalopathy syndrome (PRES)**
    - Edema in the posterior region of the brain due to failure of local blood pressure regulation at the capillary level usually due to systemic insult including hypertension, autoimmune disease, or other illness.
    - Most common type of PRES seizure is Tonic clonic
  - **PRES**
    - In addition to seizures, other symptoms include visual disturbances sush as homonymous hemianopsia and cortical blindness, as well as mild confusion, agitation or coma
  - **Eclampsia**
    - Signs: Hypertension >140/90, tonic-clonic seizure.
    - Symptoms: headache, epigastric pain, visual changes, pulmonary edema, oliguria.
    - Definitive treatment is delivery of fetus.
    - Prophylaxis with magnesium.

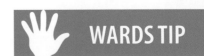

**WARDS TIP**

PRES is most commonly associated with severe hypertension in the setting of eclampsia or renal failure. Vasogenic edema contributes to severe headache and visual disturbance.

**TABLE 10-1. Antiepileptic Drugs (AEDs)**

| Epilepsy Drugs | Partial (Focal) | Generalized | | Status Epilepticus | Mechanism | Side Effects | Notes |
|---|---|---|---|---|---|---|---|
| | | Tonic-Clonic | Absence | | | | |
| Ethosuximide | | | ✓[a] | | Blocks thalamic T-type $Ca^{2+}$ channels | **EFGHIJ**—Ethosuximide causes **F**atigue, **G**I distress, **H**eadache, **I**tching (and urticaria), and Stevens-**J**ohnson syndrome | **S**ucks to have **S**ilent (absence) **S**eizures |
| Benzodiazepines (eg, diazepam, lorazepam, midazolam) | | | | ✓[b] | ↑$GABA_A$ action | Sedation, tolerance, dependence, respiratory depression | Also for eclampsia seizures (first line is $MgSO_4$) |
| Phenobarbital | ✓ | ✓ | | | ↑$GABA_A$ action | Sedation, tolerance, dependence, induction of cytochrome P-450, cardiorespiratory depression | First line in neonates |
| Phenytoin, fosphenytoin | ✓ | ✓[a] | | ✓[c] | Blocks $Na^+$ channels; zero-order kinetics | Neurologic: nystagmus, diplopia, ataxia, sedation, peripheral neuropathy. Dermatologic: hirsutism, Stevens-Johnson syndrome, gingival hyperplasia, DRESS syndrome. Musculoskeletal: osteopenia, SLE-like syndrome. Hematologic: megaloblastic anemia. Reproductive: teratogenesis (fetal hydantoin syndrome). Other: cytochrome P-450 induction | |
| Carbamazepine | ✓[a] | ✓ | | | Blocks $Na^+$ channels | Diplopia, ataxia, blood dyscrasias (agranulocytosis, aplastic anemia), liver toxicity, teratogenesis, induction of cytochrome P-450, SIADH, Stevens-Johnson syndrome | First line for trigeminal neuralgia |
| Valproic acid | ✓ | ✓[a] | ✓ | | ↑$Na^+$ channel inactivation, ↑GABA concentration by inhibiting GABA transaminase | GI distress, rare but fatal hepatotoxicity (measure LFTs), pancreatitis, neural tube defects, tremor, weight gain, contraindicated in pregnancy | Also used for myoclonic seizures, bipolar disorder, migraine prophylaxis |
| Vigabatrin | ✓ | | | | ↑GABA by irreversibly inhibiting GABA transaminase | Permanent visual loss (black box warning) | |
| Gabapentin | ✓ | | | | Primarily inhibits high-voltage-activated $Ca^{2+}$ channels; designed as GABA analog | Sedation, ataxia | Also used for peripheral neuropathy, postherpetic neuralgia |
| Topiramate | ✓ | ✓ | | | Blocks $Na^+$ channels, ↑GABA | Sedation, mental dulling, kidney stones, weight loss, glaucoma | |
| Lamotrigine | ✓ | ✓ | ✓ | | Blocks voltage-gated $Na^+$ channels, inhibits the release of glutamate | Stevens-Johnson syndrome (must be titrated slowly) | |
| Levetiracetam | ✓ | ✓ | | | Unknown; may modulate GABA and glutamate release | Fatigue, drowsiness, headache, neuropsychiatric symptoms (eg, personality changes) | |
| Tiagabine | ✓ | | | | ↑GABA by inhibiting reuptake | | |

[a]First line.
[b]First line for acute.
[c]First line for prophylaxis.

**Case 1:** A 4-year-old girl has recurrent episodes of loss of body tone, with associated falls, as well as complex partial seizures and, at times, generalized tonic-clonic seizures. Her cognitive function has been deteriorating. EEG shows 1- to 2-Hz spike-and-wave discharges. Which of the following is the most likely diagnosis?

A. Febrile seizures
B. Lennox-Gastaut syndrome
C. Juvenile myoclonic epilepsy
D. Mitochondrial encephalomyopathy
E. Landau-Kleffner syndrome

The correct answer is B. This patient suffers from Lennox-Gastaut syndrome, which is characterized by cognitive decline, multiple seizure types, and 1- to 2-Hz generalized spike-wave discharges on EEG. Many patients exhibit infantile spasms (West syndrome). Infants and children with infantile spasms exhibit paroxysmal flexions of the body, waist, or neck and usually have a profoundly disorganized EEG pattern called hypsarrhythmia.

**Case 2:** A 36-year-old man develops involuntary twitching movements in his right thumb. Within 30 seconds, he notices that the twitching has spread to his entire right hand and that involuntary movements have developed in his right forearm and the right side of his face. He cannot recall what happened subsequently, but his fiancé reports that he fell to the floor and the entire right side of his body appeared stiffened and then seemed to be twitching rhythmically. He appeared to be unresponsive for about 3 minutes and confused for another 45 minutes. During the episode, he bit his tongue and lost his urine. What is his diagnosis?

A. Jacksonian march leading to a generalized tonic-clonic seizure
B. Romberg
C. Complex—partial seizure
D. Myoclonic seizure

The correct answer is A. Jacksonian march leading to a generalized tonic-clonic seizure. A Jacksonian march is where a simple partial motor seizure spreads from the distal limb. As the seizure spreads along the motor strip in the brain, there is a "march" of the motor symptoms.

**Case 3:** A 5-year-old boy has frequent staring spells and does not respond when his mother calls his name during these episodes. He never falls down or bites his tongue. EEG reveals a 3-Hz spike-and-wave pattern that occurs for less than 10 seconds at a time but several times an hour. The child has normal motor and cognitive development but has recently been sent to the principal's office for not "paying attention" in class. The treatment of choice is:

A. Divalproex
B. Ethosuximide
C. Phenytoin
D. Ativan
E. Pentobarbital

The correct answer is B. Ethosuximide is used to treat absence seizures.

**NOTES**

# CHAPTER 11

# HEADACHE DISORDERS

In this chapter, we will review the topic of headache, which is the most common symptom encountered by neurologists. Pain is caused by irritation to structures in the head and neck such as the dura, cranial nerves (particularly the trigeminal nerve), and muscles. A careful and thorough history is necessary to distinguish *primary* and *secondary* causes of headache.

## Headache History

Taking a history in a patient with headache should focus on the following key points:

- Onset
- Time to peak (ie, sudden onset or gradually worsening)
- Location and laterality
- Quality of the pain (ie, throbbing, stabbing, pressure, pulsating)
- Duration
- Alleviating and aggravating factors
- Associated symptoms
- Key: inquire if this is a new headache or like headaches the patient has experienced in the past

## Primary Headache

The most common primary headache disorders include migraine, tension-type headache, and trigeminal autonomic cephalgias such as cluster headache and trigeminal neuralgia.

### MIGRAINE

Migraine is one of the most prevalent primary headache disorders, second only to tension-type headaches.

- Classic Migraine - has aura
- Common Migrane - does not have aura
- More common in females.
- Unilateral, pulsating, or throbbing headaches that last 4 to 72 hours and are associated with nausea and/or vomiting, photophobia, or phonophobia.
- Headaches are worsened by routine physical activity.

Migraine is divided into five phases:

- **Prodrome:** Initial symptoms including yawning, cravings, polyuria, mood changes, irritability, light sensitivity, neck pain, and cognitive dysfunction that precede headache or aura by up to 48 hours.
- **Aura:** Transient visual, sensory, motor, language, or brainstem signs, lasting 5 to 60 minutes that may precede, occur during, or occur without the headache phase of migraine.
  - Occurs in about one-third of patients with migraine.
  - Visual aura may consist of field cuts, obscurations, and scotoma and typically marches across the visual field over 15 to 20 minutes. Common visual auras include a scintillating scotoma or fortification scotoma.
- **Headache:** The hallmark of migraine, thought to be secondary to activation of trigeminal nociceptors. Pain is due to release of substance P, calcitonin gene-related peptide (CGRP), nitric oxide, and vasoactive peptides.

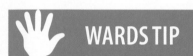

**WARDS TIP**

Migraine headaches are associated with nausea/vomiting and/or photophobia/phonophobia. They are worsened by routine physical activity and are often debilitating.

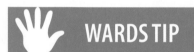

**WARDS TIP**

The diagnosis of migraine requires at least five headache attacks meeting migraine criteria.

Headache phase of migraine is debilitating; most patients withdraw to a quiet, dark room.

- **Postdrome:** Nonheadache symptoms, including fatigue and poor concentration in the 24 to 48 hours following resolution of headaches.

- **Interictal:** Relatively symptom-free period between migraine attacks. Patients can experience hypersensitivity, autonomic symptoms, and cognitive dysfunction during this period.

There are several recognized variants of migraine:

- **Familial hemiplegic migraine:** Migraine with aura associated with specific gene mutations, where aura consists of fully reversible motor weakness and/or fully reversible visual, sensory, and/or speech/language symptoms. Weakness typically lasts up to 72 hours.

- **Abdominal migraine:** Recurrent attacks of moderate to severe, midline abdominal pain *without headache* associated with nausea and vomiting, pallor, or anorexia lasting up to 72 hours. Primarily seen in children.

- **Retinal migraine:** Recurrent attacks of monocular vision loss or visual disturbances associated with migraine headache. Must exclude other causes of transient visual loss or amaurosis fugax.

Complications of migraine include:

- **Status migrainosis:** Intractable migraine attack lasting at least 72 hours.

- **Stroke:** There is a twofold increased risk of ischemic stroke in patients with migraine with aura. Stroke may also occur during a migraine with aura attack, causing prolonged aura symptoms.

**Treatment of migraine** includes abortive treatments for an acute attack and prophylactic treatments to reduce attack frequency.

- Prophylaxis: Lifestyle changes (sleep hygiene, exercise, diet), beta-blockers (propranolol; do not use in patients with asthma or COPD), anticonvulsants (topiramate, caution in patients with nephrolithiasis; valproate), calcium channel blockers (verapamil), tricyclic antidepressants (amitriptyline).
  - Newer agents include CGRP antagonists (erenumab, fremanezumab, galcanezumab, eptinezumab).

- Abortive: Triptans (5-hydroxytryptamine 1B, 1D, and 1F agonists such as sumatriptan, caution in patients with history of coronary artery disease or stroke), dihydroergotamine; antiemetics can be used as adjuvant treatment.

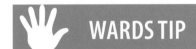

**WARDS TIP**

Prophylactic migraine therapy is considered when a patient has at least 6 to 8 headache days per month. An adequate trial of a prophylactic headache medication takes 30 days.

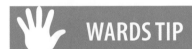

**WARDS TIP**

Triptans are most effective when administered early in a migraine attack.

## TENSION-TYPE HEADACHES

**Tension-type headaches** are the most common type of primary headache.

- Bilateral, mild to moderate in intensity, and last minutes to days.
- Often described as "band-like" pain around the head.
- In contrast to migraine, pain does not worsen with routine activity and is not associated with nausea.
- **Treatment:** NSAIDs, acetaminophen; amitriptyline for chronic pain.

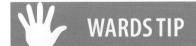

**WARDS TIP**

Unlike migraine, tension-type headaches do not interfere with daily activities.

## CLUSTER HEADACHES

Trigeminal pain with prominent autonomic features (Table 11-1).

■Epidemiology: More common in males with peak incidence 20 to 50 years old.

- Risk factors: Smoking and **passive smoke** exposure, prior head trauma, and genetics.

## TABLE 11-1. Comparison of Migraine, Tension, and Cluster Headache

| Headache Type | Location | Duration | Description and Associated Symptoms | Treatment |
|---|---|---|---|---|
| **Migraine** | Unilateral | 4-72 hours | Pulsating or **throbbing** pain with nausea, **photophobia**, or phonophobia. May have aura. Pain worsens with routine physical activity. | Acute: triptans, dihydroergotamine, antiemetics<br>Chronic: lifestyle changes, propranolol, verapamil, amitriptyline, topiramate, valproate, CGRP antagonists |
| **Tension** | Bilateral | >30 minutes to 7 days | Steady, "band-like" pain without aura or nausea. Pain does not worsen with routine physical activity. | Acute: NSAIDs, acetaminophen<br>Chronic: amitriptyline |
| **Cluster** | Unilateral | 15 minutes to 3 hours; recurrent attacks daily or every other day for weeks to months followed by periods of remission for months to years | Excruciating frontal, temporal, or periorbital pain with lacrimation, rhinorrhea, eyelid edema. May present with Horner's syndrome. Associated with agitation or **restless**ness. | Acute: sumatriptan, 100% O$_2$<br>Chronic: verapamil |

**WARDS TIP**

The key features of cluster headache can be remembered with the mnemonic **SEAR**:
**S**ide locked
**E**xcruciating
**A**gitating
**R**egularly recurring attacks

**WARDS TIP**

Unlike patients with migraine, patients with cluster headache cannot go lie down in a dark, quiet room and often feel a sense of restlessness or agitation.

**KEY FACT**

Cluster headaches are unilateral and always associated with autonomic symptoms.

**WARDS TIP**

Stop prophylactic medication for cluster headache 2 weeks after an attack cycle ends to prevent tachyphylaxis.

- Presentation: Severe, unilateral frontal, temporal, or periorbital pain.
  - As a rule, headache is side locked in cluster headache but *can switch sides* between attacks or within a cycle.
  - Associated with unilateral **autonomic symptoms**, including lacrimation, rhinorrhea, or nasal congestion, miosis, ptosis, eyelid edema, or conjunctival injection occurring on the same side as headache pain.
    - Can be associated with **Horner's syndrome.**
  - Headaches occur with periodicity in cycles lasting weeks to month with up to eight attacks per day, each lasting 15 minutes to 3 hours followed by periods of remission lasting months to years.
  - Headaches can wake patients from sleep, often at the same time each night shortly after sleep onset.
- Treatment includes prophylaxis and abortive strategies:
  - Prophylaxis: Channel blockers (verapamil, can cause severe constipation).
  - Abortive: 100% oxygen, triptans.

## TRIGEMINAL NEURALGIA (TIC DOULOUREUX)

- Brief paroxysms lasting <1 minute of severe, lancinating (electric shock-like, shooting, stabbing, sharp) pain in the distribution of the trigeminal nerve.
- Most commonly affects V2 (maxillary) or V3 (mandibular) divisions. Less likely to affect V1 (ophthalmic) division.
- Can be triggered by chewing, eating, talking, light touch over the face, brushing teeth.
- Often idiopathic. Suspect a secondary cause especially if symptoms are bilateral or there are pronounced sensory changes.
  - Secondary causes include compression of the trigeminal nerve by a vascular loop and multiple sclerosis.
- Treatment: Carbamazepine or oxcarbazepine. Surgical decompression of vascular loop.

## Secondary Headache

Secondary headaches are headaches associated with another disorder known to cause headache. It is essential to distinguish secondary headaches from primary headaches to exclude treatable or life-threatening causes.

Red flags that suggest a secondary cause of headache (and reasons to obtain neuroimaging) can be remembered with the mnemonic **SNOOP4**:

- **S**ystemic symptoms and **S**econdary risk factors: fever, night sweats, chills, weight loss, jaw claudication; cancer, immunocompromised or immunosuppressed states, chronic infection
- **N**eurologic signs/symptoms: confusion, focal neurologic deficits, pulsatile tinnitus
- **O**nset: thunderclap
- **O**lder age: new or progressive headache after age >50
- **P**ositional: headache worsens with change in position
- **P**rior history: new onset or change to persistent headache
- **P**regnancy: new-onset headache during pregnancy
- **P**recipitated by Valsalva maneuvers: headache precipitated by coughing, sneezing, bending over, straining (results in increased intracranial pressure [ICP])

### IDIOPATHIC INTRACRANIAL HYPERTENSION (IIH; PSEUDOTUMOR CEREBRI)

Idiopathic intracranial hypertension is a headache disorder characterized by elevated ICP without an identifiable cause.

Key clinical features are related to high ICP:
- Holocephalic headache
- Worsening headache when supine, improvement when upright
- **Transient visual changes**
- Pulsatile tinnitus
- **Papilledema**
- Diplopia (due to CN VI palsy)
- Peripheral visual loss followed by central vision loss

Risk factors and epidemiology:
- **Female sex**
- Peak incidence 20 to 30 years old
- Obesity
- Medications: that can cause vitamin A, oral contraceptives, tetracycline, corticosteroids
- Diagnosis is made by observing an **elevated opening pressure** >250 mm CSF (25 cm H2O) on lumbar puncture without an identifiable lesion.
- CSF profile is otherwise normal.
- Neuroimaging does not demonstrate hydrocephalus or mass lesion.

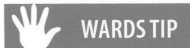

**WARDS TIP**

Loss of sensation should not be present with trigeminal neuralgia.

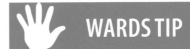

**WARDS TIP**

Bilateral trigeminal neuralgia should raise concern for a secondary cause.

**WARDS TIP**

Anyone presenting with a new single headache rather than recurrent headaches should be evaluated for secondary causes of headache.

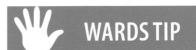

**WARDS TIP**

The most important complication of IIH is vision loss due to compressive optic neuropathy. Goal of treatment is to lower ICP to prevent vision loss.

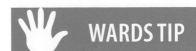

**WARDS TIP**

Venous sinus thrombosis may mimic IIH and should always be excluded with venous imaging.

Treatment:

- Carbonic anhydrase inhibitors: acetazolamide, topiramate
- CSF shunting
- Therapeutic lumbar puncture
- Optic nerve sheath fenestration

## INTRACRANIAL HYPOTENSION

Headache that develops spontaneously or following minor trauma, lumbar puncture, or strenuous physical activity that results in CSF leakage out of the subarachnoid space.

- Epidemiology: More common in females with peak incidence 30 to 50 years old.
- Presentation: Headaches are typically bilateral and may have migrainous features.
  - Headaches are "orthostatic," characteristically **worsening in the upright** position and improving when supine.
  - Headaches worsen with Valsalva maneuvers.
  - Additional features may include dizziness, hypoacusis, and tinnitus.
- Diagnosis
  - Brain imaging may show brain sagging or pachymeningeal enhancement.
  - CT myelography can visualize CSF leak.
- Treatment
  - Bedrest
  - Aggressive fluid repletion
  - Caffeine
  - Epidural blood patch
  - Surgical dural repair

## WORST HEADACHE OF LIFE

Patients who present with "worst headache of life" or a *thunderclap* headache should be evaluated for several key and dangerous causes of secondary headache. Thunderclap headaches are those that begin suddenly and reach peak intensity within seconds of onset.

Important causes:

- **Subarachnoid hemorrhage:** Obtain CT head without contrast to look for presence of subarachnoid blood. Lumbar puncture can be done to evaluate for xanthochromia and presence of red blood cells.
- **Reversible cerebral vasoconstriction syndrome (RCVS):** Reversible narrowing of cerebral vessels associated with SSRIs and over-the-counter cold medications such as pseudoephedrine.
- **Posterior reversible encephalopathy syndrome (PRES):** Syndrome characterized by vasogenic edema of the cerebral white matter primarily affecting the occipital and parietal lobes associated with headache, seizures, altered mental status, and visual loss.
- **Cortical venous sinus thrombosis:** Occlusion of a venous sinus, preventing drainage and causing headache and possibly focal neurologic deficits secondary to ischemic and/or hemorrhagic infarct.

---

**WARDS TIP**

Orienting the bevel of the spinal needle during LP parallel to the long axis of the spinal cord can help prevent CSF leak by minimizing trauma to the dura.

---

**WARDS TIP**

Thunderclap headaches begin suddenly and reach peak intensity in seconds. Can be associated with subarachnoid hemorrhage.

# GIANT CELL (TEMPORAL) ARTERITIS (GCA)

- Systemic granulomatous inflammation of medium and large vessels, most commonly involving branches of the carotid artery, especially the temporal artery.
- Epidemiology: More common in **females** and typically occurs over age 50 with mean age 70 years old.
- Presentation: Unilateral or bilateral headache associated with vision loss, jaw claudication, fever, weight loss, fatigue, **scalp tenderness**, or palpable nodularity of the temporal artery.
  - Can be associated with polymyalgia rheumatica (PMR).
  - Severely affected vessels may thrombose, resulting in stroke and lead to vision loss.
- Diagnosis
  - Elevated erythrocyte sedimentation rate (**ESR**).
  - Temporal artery ultrasound may demonstrate "halo sign."
  - Temporal artery biopsy: Vasculitis and granulomatous inflammation.
- Treatment: High-dose corticosteroids.

## WARDS TIP

Consider GCA on the differential in all patients over 50 years old with a new headache.

## KEY FACT

The most worrisome complication of GCA is vision loss due to anterior ischemic optic neuropathy. Prompt diagnosis and treatment is essential.

## KEY FACT

When GCA is associated with stroke, it is commonly associated with posterior circulation infarcts.

**Case 1:** A 28-year-old male smoker with a history of a concussion presents with severe left-sided headache. He describes stabbing pain radiating from his left temple toward his forehead associated with left-sided nasal drainage, eyelid swelling, and conjunctival injection. He often is woken up by headaches at night. He feels agitated and anxious during the headache and cannot sit still. Ibuprofen and Tylenol do not help. He often experiences multiple headaches a day, each lasting 2 hours, and notes these headaches tend to occur during the spring and fall months. What is this patient's diagnosis?

A. Migraine headache
B. Cluster headache
C. Tension headache
D. Headache secondary to Giant Cell Arteritis

The correct answer is B. This patient's severe, unilateral pain associated with rhinorrhea, eyelid swelling, and conjunctival injection is consistent with cluster headache, characterized by trigeminal pain with prominent autonomic features. These tend to occur with periodicity, clustering (as the name suggests) around certain times of day (shortly after sleep onset, midmorning, midafternoon, late evening) and times of year (often spring and fall). In contrast to migraine, cluster headaches are more common in men, and attacks are typically shorter in duration and autonomic symptoms are more notable. Patients with migraine classically lie down in a dark, quiet room during attacks as opposed to patients with cluster headache who feel a sense of agitation and restlessness and are unable to sit still.

***What are the treatment options in the acute setting?***

A. Triptans and high-flow oxygen
B. Calcium Channel Blocker
C. Ibuprofen
D. Ergotamine

As in migraine, there are both prophylactic and abortive treatments for cluster headache. Calcium channel blockers such as verapamil are commonly used for prophylaxis. Subcutaneous sumatriptan and high-flow oxygen are used for acute headache attacks.

**Case 2:** A 26-year-old obese woman with acne, who just started a new medication for her acne, presents with 2 months of headache. She describes worsening pain with lying flat, coughing, and straining. She describes holocephalic pain and intermittent, transient visual obscuration. She also endorses pulsatile tinnitus.

Examination should include a fundoscopic exam to look for papilledema, which is a sign of increased intracranial pressure.

***What is the likely diagnosis?***

A. Idiopathic intracranial hypertension
B. Migraine Headache
C. Cluster headache
D. Trigeminal Neuralgia.

The correct answer is a. idiopathic intracranial hypertension
This patient likely has idiopathic intracranial hypertension (IIH), which is most commonly seen in young, obese women. IIH is associated with obesity and certain medications, including vitamin A derivatives and tetracyclines such as those used to treat acne and oral contraceptives. Corticosteroids are also associated with IIH. Next step in diagnosis would include neuroimaging and performing a lumbar puncture and measuring the opening pressure. The patient is at risk for vision loss. Classically, IIH is associated with peripheral visual loss followed by central vision loss.

**Case 3:** A 45-year-old man comes to the emergency department 4 hours after the sudden onset of a severe headache. The pain is associated with nausea and vomiting. Medical history is noncontributory. He is drowsy but easily aroused. His temperature is 37.3°C (98.2°F), pulse is 88/min, respirations are 11/min, and blood pressure is 140/70 mm Hg. Examination of the head shows no external injuries. Flexion of the neck produces pain. The optic fundi are normal. Motor and sensory examinations show no abnormalities. Cranial nerves are intact. Deep tendon reflexes are symmetric. Babinski sign is present bilaterally. Which of the following is most likely to confirm the diagnosis?

A. X-rays of the sinuses
B. Carotid duplex ultrasonography
C. EEG
D. CT scan of the head
E. Biopsy of the temporal artery

The correct answer is D. This patient is presenting with sudden severe headache, with signs of elevated ICP including drowsiness, nausea and vomiting, and positive Babinski sign. Neck stiffness is meningismus due to SAH blood irritating the meninges. An intracerebral hemorrhage or subarachnoid hemorrhage should be ruled out with CT scan of the head as initial workup.

# CHAPTER 12

# NEOPLASTIC DISORDERS

The focus of this chapter is to provide you with a general overview of tumors involving the nervous system. It will be important to know their prognosis and treatment options.

Also, keep in mind some of the "buzz-words" that describe histopathological hallmarks of each type of tumor.

## Primary CNS Tumors

Metastatic brain tumors are 10 times more common than primary malignant brain tumors and therefore the most common brain tumor overall.

### PILOCYTIC ASTROCYTOMA (PA)

- *Patients*: more common in *childhood*
- *Location*: cerebellum, optic chiasm (associated with NF1), hypothalamus, periventricular
- *Imaging*: enhancing mural nodule with a cystic component
- *Microscopy*: pilocytic elongated cells, **Rosenthal fibers** (Fig. 12-1)
- *Treatment*: surgical resection

### GLIOBLASTOMA MULTIFORME

- *Patients*: adults (peak incidence—64-year-old)
- *Location*: cerebral hemispheres
- *Imaging*: heterogeneously enhancing lesion with vasogenic edema and necrotic core; may cross midline (butterfly glioma)
- *Microscopy*: **pseudopalisading** with necrosis
- *Treatment*: radiation and chemotherapy (temozolomide), resection to delay disease progression

### OLIGODENDROGLIOMA

- *Patients*: adults (around age 40)
- *Location*: frontal lobes (seizures, personality change)

**KEY FACT**

Optic glioma is a grade 1 PA that arises from glial cells of optic pathway. Surgical resection if symptomatic; radiotherapy if unresectable. Patients will continue to have visual impairment.

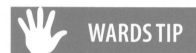

**WARDS TIP**

GBM is a fast growing and invasive brain tumor. More common in men, survival is less than 20% after 2 years.

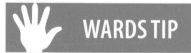

**WARDS TIP**

GBM is the most common form of malignant primary brain tumor.

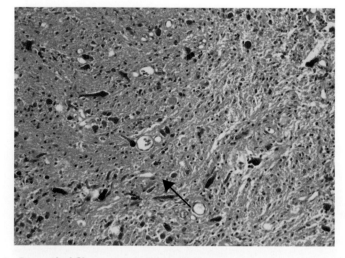

**FIGURE 12-1. Rosenthal fibers seen in Pilocytic Astrocytoma.** Reproduced with permission from Kemp WL, Burns DK, Brow TG: *Pathology: The Big Picture*. New York, NY: McGraw Hill; 2008.

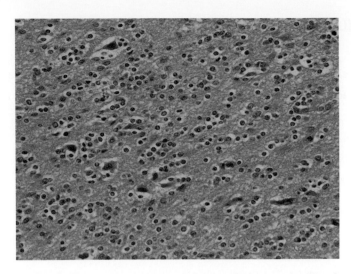

**FIGURE 12-2.** **"Fried egg" appearance with clear cytoplasm seen in oligodendroglioma.** (Used with permission from Dr. Stephen Cohle, *Spectrum Health-Blodgett Campus,* Grand Rapids, MI.)

- *Imaging*: variable
- *Microscopy*: "**fried egg**" appearance with clear cytoplasm (Fig. 12-2)
- *Treatment*: resection and radiation

## EPENDYMOMA

- *Patients*: more common in children, associated with NF2
- *Location*: posterior fossa/ventricular system (children), spinal cord (adults) arises from ependymal lining of ventricles
- *Imaging*:
  - Intracranial tumors—heterogeneous, slightly enhancing
  - Spinal tumors—homogeneous, brightly enhancing
- *Microscopy*: **perivascular pseudorosettes**, GFAP+ (Fig. 12-3)
- *Treatment*: resection

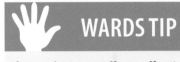

**WARDS TIP**

If ependymoma affects affecting ventricular system, expect non-communicating hydrocephalus.

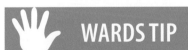

**WARDS TIP**

*Von Hippel-Lindau syndrome is an autosomal dominant cancer syndrome associated with cerebellar and spinal cord hemangioblastomas, renal cell carcinoma, pheochromocytoma, and retinal angiomas.*

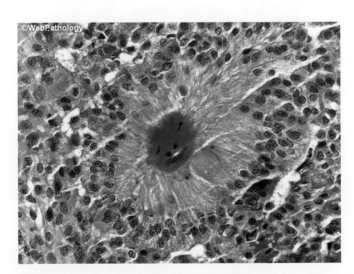

**FIGURE 12-3.** **Perivascular pseudorosettes seen in Ependymoma.** WebPathology

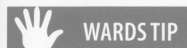

*Hemangiomas can produce erythropoietin, causing secondary polycythemia.*

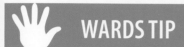

*Patients undergoing resection of craniopharyngioma can have complications including vision changes, hypothalamic injury, and diabetes insipidus.*

**KEY FACT**

Tumor cells synthesize erythropoietin > secondary polycythemia.

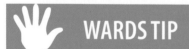

Treat prolactinoma with dopamine agonists (cabergoline, bromocriptine).

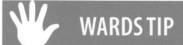

Pituitary apoplexy: macroadenoma that outgrows or compresses the blood supply causing hemorrhage. Can lead to severe acute onset headache and visual impairment.

## HEMANGIOBLASTOMA

- *Patients*:
  - Associated with von Hippel-Lindau disease—children, young adults
  - Sporadic—adulthood
- *Location*: cerebellum, spinal cord
- *Imaging*: cyst with enhancing mural nodule
- *Microscopy*: vascular tumor
- *Treatment*: resection

## MENINGIOMA

- *Patients*: older adults, female predominance; associated with radiation exposure and NF2
- *Location*: cerebral convexities
- *Imaging*: extra-axial lesion with dural tail of enhancement (Fig. 12-4)
- *Microscopy*: whorls and **psammoma bodies**
- *Treatment*: resection; radiation if anaplastic, recurrent, or inoperable

## PITUITARY ADENOMA

- *Patients*: headache, bitemporal hemianopia, and potentially endocrinological complaints, Multiple Endocrine Neoplasia (MEN) Type 1 (symptoms dependent on tumor size due to mass effect and secretion status)
- *Microscopy*: classification based on immunostaining for hormones
- *Treatment*: medical management of endocrinopathies, resection, radiation for recurrence

## SCHWANNOMA

- *Patients*: cranial nerve 5, 7, 8 and 9 compression/dysfunction (hearing loss, dysequilibrium, facial weakness, or sensory change)
  - Bilateral vestibular schwannomas are associated with NF2
- *Location*: cerebellopontine angle

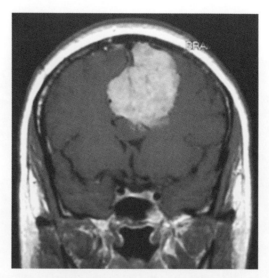

**FIGURE 12-4. Extra-axial lesion at midline consistent with meningioma.** Reproduced with permission from Allan H. Ropper, Martin A. Samuels, Joshua P. Klein, Sashank Prasad, *Adams and Victor's Principles of Neurology, 11ed*. Fig 30-7. McGraw-Hill. ISBN 9780071842617

- *Imaging*: well-circumscribed mass with fatty and/or cystic components
- *Microscopy*: **Verocay bodies** (linear palisades of nuclei)
- *Treatment*: resection

## MEDULLOBLASTOMA

- *Patients*: most common in children; present with headaches, vomiting, and vision changes (signs of obstructive hydrocephalus) as well as broad-based gait or truncal ataxia (cerebellar involvement)
- *Location*: midline cerebellum or vermis
- *Imaging*: hyperintense on T2 with heterogeneous enhancement
- *Microscopy*: small, round, blue cells with **Homer Wright rosettes**
- *Treatment*: resection and radiation

## CRANIOPHARYNGIOMA

- *Patients*:
  - Bimodal distribution: children 5 to 15 and adults 45 to 60
  - Presentation: endocrinopathy, bitemporal hemianopia
- *Location*: sellar region
- *Imaging*: cystic suprasellar mass with enhancing cystic components
- *Microscopy*: adamantinomatous or papillary variants
  - Cholesterol crystals are pathognomonic for adamantinomatous variant
- *Treatment*: resection, radiation, and/or hormone replacement therapy

## PRIMARY CNS LYMPHOMA

- *Patients*: increased risk in HIV/AIDS patients (CD4 < 100), elderly
- *Location*: periventricular, diencephalon
- *Imaging*: solitary ring-enhancing lesion
- *Microscopy*: polymorphous large cells that have B-cell markers (CD 4, 19, 20, 22, 79a)
- *Treatment*: chemotherapy (high-dose methotrexate), antiretroviral therapy for HIV

## Metastatic CNS Tumors

## BRAIN

- Most common brain tumor in adults
  - Primary malignancy: lung, breast > melanoma, renal cell, thyroid
  - Up to three-fourth of patients have multiple lesions at presentation
  - Predilection for **gray-white junction** or watershed areas due to vascular/endothelial spread
- Presentation: depends on location and amount of edema
  - Signs of elevated intracranial pressure—headache, vomiting, altered mental status
  - Focal deficits—weakness, vision changes, seizures, speech changes
  - Treatment: whole-body contrast CT, PET scan, or brain biopsy to determine primary tumor type

**KEY FACT**

Turcot syndrome = medulloblastoma + familial adenomatous polyposis

**KEY FACT**

Rathke's cleft cysts similar in presentation to craniopharyngiomas. The difference is that craniopharyngiomas grow by cell division and fluid accumulation, whereas Rathke's cleft cysts grow only by fluid accumulation.

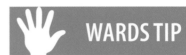

**WARDS TIP**

*Radiation therapy can have many complications, including encephalopathy, myelopathy, cognitive impairment, cranial neuropathies, and radiation necrosis. These complications may be delayed by months after treatment.*

- Prophylactic radiation (stereotactic radiosurgery or whole-brain, depending on tumor burden) and/or chemotherapy
- Surgical resection has the best outcome for young patients with good performance status, limited systemic disease, and a single metastatic lesion
■ Symptom management:
- Antiepileptic therapies are not recommended as prophylaxis, but should be considered if seizures are present
  - Must use caution to avoid antiepileptics that can impact chemotherapy metabolism
- Corticosteroids can help with edema
■ Survival varies but is typically months

## LEPTOMENINGEAL

■ Rare complication of advanced solid tumor cancers (breast, lung, melanoma)
■ Multifocal involvement is hallmark as it affects multiple regions of craniospinal axis
■ Diagnosis: Leptomeningeal enhancement on MRI, abnormal CSF analysis

## SPINAL CORD

■ Can be extradural, intradural, intramedullary (within the cord)
■ Most commonly seen in breast, prostate, and lung cancer
■ Can occur via hematogenous spread or direct extension
■ Presentation: pain, followed by weakness and sensory changes
■ Treatment: radiation and chemotherapy
■ Symptom management:
- Pain management
- Corticosteroids, especially if weakness is present

**Case 1:** A 29-year-old man has headaches upon awakening. MRI shows a brain mass. Which of the following is the most common source of primary brain tumors?

A. Lymphocytes
B. Glial cells
C. Meningeal cells
D. Endothelial cells
E. Neurons

The correct answer is B. The most common primary brain tumor is the astrocytoma, which is derived from glial cells.

**Case 2:** At his annual physical examination by his pediatrician, an 8-year-old boy is discovered to have precocious puberty. More careful examination discovers the presence of papilledema and difficulty with looking upwards. This patient is most likely to have which of the following?

A. Ependymoma
B. Oligodendroglioma
C. Brainstem glioma
D. Astrocytoma
E. Pituitary adenoma

The correct answer is E. pituitary gland tumors that can cause hormone release, increased intracranial pressure, as well as Parinaud's syndrome where there is difficulty with upgaze.

**Case 3:** A 23-year-old woman who uses a tanning bed regularly develops malignant melanoma. This is discovered not during skin exam but as part of the workup for new-onset headaches and confusion, when MRI brain showed multiple small hemorrhages. Metastatic lesions to the brain most often appear in which of the following locations?

A. In the sella turcica
B. In the caudate
C. In the posterior fossa
D. In the thalamus
E. At the gray-white junction

The correct answer is E. Metastatic lesions are spread primarily by the vascular system. The gray-white junction is the location at which blood-borne cancer cells are most likely to lodge and grow.

**NOTES**

# EMBRYOLOGY AND
# CONGENITAL DISORDERS

This chapter provides you with the highest yield information on the development of the nervous system as well as disorders that arise during this process. It will be important to be familiar with the various congenital diseases, their genetic basis (if there is one), and the treatment and management of each.

## Embryology and Development of the Nervous System

Development of the nervous system fits into the larger process of creating the whole person from a fertilized egg. Disruptions of development create predictable neurologic syndromes.

■ Week 3-4: Neurulation—After gastrulation, the mesoderm develops the notochord which *induces the ectoderm* to differentiate into nervous system tissue (neural plate) (Fig. 13-1).
  • Neuronal stem cells accumulate on the neural plate over the notochord which begins to fold as the weight of the cells increases, becoming a groove, then a fold, and then a tube.
  • By the 28th day after fertilization, there is a neural tube (derived from the ectoderm) surrounded by somites (mesodermal structures that will become the bony spinal cord and paraspinus muscles).
  • The neural fold zips itself up (becomes a true tube) from the middle toward the top and bottom simultaneously.
  • Folate is necessary for this process to occur, which is why all prenatal vitamins contain folate.

### NEUROLOGIC DEVELOPMENT

■ Week 4-5:
  • Brain development—Once the cranial neuropore is closed, the developing nervous system divides into three primary and five secondary vesicles (Table 13.1).
  • Spinal cord development—Cells of the developing spinal cord produce two separate plates.
    – Dorsally, the Alar plate will have all the sensory neurons.
    – Ventrally, the Basal plate will have all the motor neurons.
    – Some neurons migrate to the intermediolateral cell column to form the autonomic nervous system, and some move to the edges to become the peripheral ganglia (ie, the dorsal root ganglia).

Almost all *brain tumors arise from neuronal stem cells* (such as Primitive Neuronal Ectodermal Tumors—PNETs), glial cells (eg, astrocytomas, oligodendroglimos, and glioblastoma multiforme), ependymal cells (eg, ependymomas), meninges (eg, meningiomas), and neuronal glandular tissue (eg, pituitary adenomas).

## KEY FACT

Week **4**—Nervous system develops through **four** discrete stages = **neural plate → neural groove → neural fold → neural tube**

## WARDS TIP

Failure to close the cranial neuropore produces encephaloceles and anencephaly (absent brain tissue, ↑AFP).

## WARDS TIP

Failure to close the caudal neuropore produces a spectrum of disease from mild (as in spina bifida occulta) to severe (as in spina bifida aperta) aka myelomeningocele.

## KEY FACT

**5th** week, **5** vesicles

| TABLE 13-1. Neural Tube Differentiation | | | |
|---|---|---|---|
| **Embryonic Brain** | | **Adult Brain Derivative** | **Associated Ventricular Space** |
| Prosencephalon | Telencephalon | Cortex, basal ganglia, hippocampus | Lateral ventricles |
| | Diencephalon | Thalamus, hypothalamus | Third ventricle |
| Mesencephalon | | Midbrain | Cerebral aqueduct |
| Rhombencephalon | Metencephalon | Cerebellum, pons | Fourth ventricle |
| | Myelencephalon | Medulla | Fourth ventricle |
| Spinal cord | | Spinal cord | Central canal |

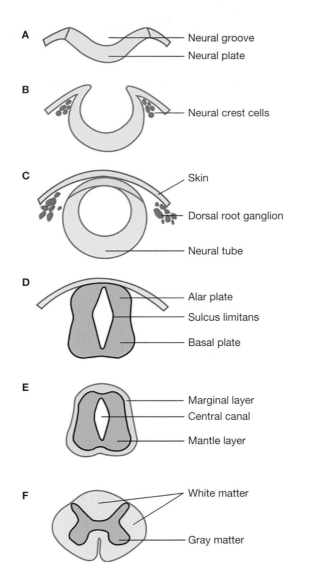

**FIGURE 13-1. Spinal cord development.** Reproduced with permission from S Waxman. *Clinical Neuroanatomy, 29e.* NY: McGraw-Hill. 2020.

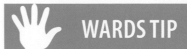 **WARDS TIP**

Failure of the telencephalon to divide into two halves produces **holoprosencephaly.**

**WARDS TIP**

The eye develops from an outgrowth of the forebrain; thus, the "optic nerve" is not a nerve at all, but an outgrowth of the central nervous system. This is why vision can be impaired in disorders of central nervous system myelin, like multiple sclerosis, but not disorders of peripheral nervous system myelin, like Guillain-Barre syndrome.

**WARDS TIP**

If you are asked on the wards what kind of tumor the patient has, "Glioma" is almost always a safe guess!

**WARDS TIP**

Folate plays an important role in closure of the neuropores, which sometimes happens before a pregnancy has been discovered. As such, everyone wishing to become pregnant is recommended to take a folate vitamin to reduce the risk of neural tube defects. Always ask about folate supplementation during health maintenance visits by patients of reproductive age.

*The Complete Nervous System*

If the above steps occur correctly, at viability (currently 23-24 weeks), the brain and spinal cord will have all the neurons they will ever have, in their final locations, and they will be in the process of developing synaptic connections. From 24 to 44 weeks, normal sulci and gyri will develop in response to the increasing weight of neuronal axons and dendrites forming these connections. Humans are born with very little myelin, probably to keep the head small enough to facilitate vaginal birth. Myelination occurs predictably over the first 5 years of life, starting at motor roots.

## Neural Tube Defects and Disorders of Early Neurologic Development

What happens when developmental anomalies occur very early in development? In this section, we look at diseases that arise from failure of closure of the neural tube.

- **Spina bifida occulta** ("closed" or "hidden" spina bifida)
  - No neural material (no neurons, no meninges) protrudes through the defect.

- May have no clinical symptoms, a "sacral dimple," "sacral pit," or "tuft of hair."
  - Even if no neurologic deficit, there could be a tract from the skin to the spinal cord that would allow bacteria in. Neurosurgery needs to *close this tract* to prevent an increased risk of infections like meningitis or myelitis.

- **Spina bifida aperta** ("open" spina bifida)
  - Neural material protrudes through the defect.
    - If just meninges, this is a meningocele.
    - If neural material, this is a myelomeningocele.
  - Commonly, the defect acts like a complete spinal cord transection at that level, resulting in *paralysis and bowel/bladder/sexual dysfunction.* Rarely can have few or minor symptoms.
  - Neurosurgery will repair the defect and safely encase the spinal cord and all its elements in the spinal column. This will not restore function but will prevent infection and further injury.

- **Anencephaly:** Complete failure of cranial neuropore closure
  - None of the prosencephalon (forebrain) will form.
  - If the diencephalon, mesencephalon, metencephalon, and myelencephalon form, the neonate may survive for a time with some ability to breathe independently.
  - If any of the lower cerebral structures do not develop, there will almost certain be spontaneous pregnancy loss or stillbirth.
  - This will be detected prenatally early in the pregnancy using ultrasound, and a plan of care will be developed with OBGYN and perinatology.

- **Cranial meningocele or encephalocele:** partial failure of cranial neuropore closure
  - Occipital encephaloceles are most common.
  - Usually, there is a moderate to severe malformation of the brain along with open defect.
  - Severe epilepsy, cerebral palsy, and intellectual disability are common. Rarely, small cranial meningoceles can have good neurologic outcomes.
    - Prenatal diagnosis is important so delivery can be done by *C-section,* ideally injury to the herniated material during delivery.

- **Holoprosencephaly:** complete closure of cranial neuropore but failure of the forebrain to divide into two halves.
- This is prenatally diagnosed, although resolution of prenatal injury may not fully define the defect.
  - Alobar holoprosencephaly—Most severe, large mono-ventricle, no midline brain structures.
  - Semilobar holoprosencephaly—Second most severe, more defined cerebral structures, some (often abnormal) midline structures such as rudimentary thalami.
  - Lobar holoprosencephaly—Least severe, nearly normal brain can sometimes be seen with fused ventricles. Outcomes range from mild to severe disability.
  - Cyclopia (one midline eye) is also common.
  - Other midline defects (cardiac defects, omphalocele, cleft lip/palette) can also be seen.

## HYDROCEPHALUS

Hydrocephalus occurs when there is excessive cerebral spinal fluid (CSF) in the head causing symptoms such as seizures, headaches, or encephalopathy.

The most important distinction when assessing hydrocephalus is whether it is "obstructive" or "nonobstructive." CSF should be produced in the lateral ventricles and flow through the foramen of Monro to the third ventricle and through the cerebral aqueduct into the fourth ventricle, and then out of the ventricular system through the paired lateral foramen of Luschka (**L**ateral **L**uschka) and the midline foramen of Magendie (**M**idline **M**agendie) to circulate around the brain and spinal cord where it is absorbed by the arachnoid granulations.

Physical blockage of this flow results in obstructive hydrocephalus, most commonly caused by bleeding or lesions and requires neurosurgery to remove the blockage or place a shunt for drainage. For example, premature babies often bleed into the ventricles, blocking the Foramen of Monro. There are important exceptions where obstructive hydrocephalus is caused by genetic conditions or congenital malformations. For example, Chiari malformations result in obstructive hydrocephalus.

Nonobstructive hydrocephalus results from overproduction or failed resorption of CSF, which then accumulates in all potential spaces inside and outside the ventricular system. Most congenital hydrocephalus is nonobstructive; for example, many congenital infections (eg, TORCH infections) result in hydrocephalus. Treatment involves either decreasing CSF production or fixing the underlying cause of arachnoid granulation dysfunction (such as curing the meningitis).

## CHIARI MALFORMATIONS

All Chiari malformations involve extension of the cerebellum more caudally than expected. The degree of descent, and whether there are associated abnormalities, defines the grade of Chiari malformation.

I. **Type 0**
   a. A relatively new term meaning the cerebellum has NOT extended below the foramen but the patient has the symptoms of Chiari malformation.
   b. The term is most frequently used when patients have a cervical syrinx, headache, and dizziness without cerebellar tonsillar herniation ("zero herniation").
II. **Type 1**
   a. The cerebellar tonsils extend below the foramen magnum.
   b. Some patients will have symptoms of headache and/or dizziness, often worse while lying down and better as the day goes on.
   c. Some patients are asymptomatic.
III. **Type 2**
   a. The cerebellar vermis extends below the foramen magnum. The medulla and fourth ventricle may also extend out of the skull.
   b. Almost always accompanied by a syrinx and commonly associated with a myelomeningocele.
      i. Frequently associated with obstructive hydrocephalus.

 **KEY FACT**

The easiest way to distinguish type of hydrocephalus is to inspect the fourth ventricle on MRI or CT scan; if the fourth ventricle is large, there is probably nonobstructive hydrocephalus. If the fourth ventricle is normal sized or small, there is probably obstructive hydrocephalus.

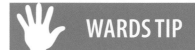 **WARDS TIP**

Only Chiari Malformation Type 2 is properly referred to as the Arnold Chiari malformation.

IV. **Type 3**
a. An uncommon diagnosis best characterized as Chiari 2 + other cerebral malformations (eg, heterotopia).

V. **Type 4**
a. Extremely uncommon and best characterized as Chiari 2 + cerebellar hypoplasia.

## PORENCEPHALY

Porencephaly occurs when a brain, otherwise well-formed, suffers injury causing tissue atrophy in utero. The result is a congenital condition in which the brain is born with a pre-existing "old" injury. Stroke is thought to be the No. 1 cause of porencephaly. Vascular malformations, congenital infection, and spontaneous hemorrhage are more-rare causes.

## Neurocutaneous Disorders

Both the skin and the nervous system derive from the ectoderm. Therefore, developmental factors that cause abnormalities in ectodermal differentiation, development, and migration might cause abnormalities in both the skin and the nervous system. Since the skin is obviously visible to the naked eye, diagnoses of specific neurologic conditions can sometimes be made merely by inspection of the skin.

## NEUROFIBROMATOSIS

- **Type 1:** Caused by mutation of *NF1* gene (neurofibromin) on Chromosome 17, a tumor suppressor gene whose mutation leads to tumors
  - Incidence: 1/4000 people (most common neurogenetic disease)
  - Skin findings: Café-au-lait spots, axillary freckling
  - Diagnostic criteria include at least two of the following:
    - Six or more café au lait > 0.5 cm in children or 1.5 cm in adults
    - Two or more neurofibromas or one plexiform neurofibroma
    - Axillary or inguinal freckling
    - Optic glioma
    - Two or more Lisch nodules
    - Bony dysplasia
    - A first-degree relative with NF1
- **Type 2:** Caused by mutation of NF2 gene (schwannomin) on Chromosome 22
  - Incidence: very rare
  - Skin findings: café-au-lait spots but usually not as many
  - Tumors on peripheral nerves, especially acoustic neuromas

## TUBEROUS SCLEROSIS

- About 80% caused by mutations on TSC1 (9q34) or TSC2 (16q13) with autosomal-dominant inheritance, but variable penetrance. The rest of the cases are thought to be caused by other, more rare, mutations of genes in the mTOR pathway.

---

**WARDS TIP**

No neurologic exam, especially in children, is complete without inspection of the skin.

---

**WARDS TIP**

NF1 and NF2 are completely different diseases and almost everyone with café-au-lait spots has NF1. NF2 is a frequent source of questions on the wards, NF2 is associated with bilateral acoustic neuroma and is a mutation of Chromosome 22.

- Incidence is rare.
- Skin findings: Ashleaf spots and Shagreen patches, adenoma sebaceum (pimple-like bumps).
- Neurologic findings: Subependymal giant cell astrocytomas (SEGA), periventricular tubers, and cortical/subcortical tubers.

## STURGE-WEBER

- Associated with GNAQ gene mutation.
- Incidence is rare.
- Skin finding: Port-wine stain in V1 distribution or broader.
  - Note: Not everyone with the port-wine stain has Sturge-Weber or an intracranial vascular malformation.
- Neurologic findings: Leptomeningeal angiomatosis (due to intracranial vascular malformation) ipsilateral to port-wine stain, strokes, seizures, and epilepsy.

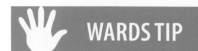

**WARDS TIP**

TSC1 and TSC2 are on chromosomes that are consecutive perfect squares; 3-squared is 9 and 4-squared is 16.

## Neurogenetic Disorders

### TRISOMIES

Sex-chromosome trisomies (XXX, XYY) produce normal phenotypes or mild disorders. Although all somatic trisomies should be equally common, only three are seen with any frequency, leading to the conclusion that all somatic trisomies except the following result in an embryonic-lethal phenotype.

*Patau Syndrome* (Chromosome 13)

- Rare
- Neurologic features: Severe intellectual disability, seizures, hypotonia, microcephaly, deafness
- Non-neurologic features: Cleft lip/palate, polydactyly, small jaw, low ears
- Typical lifespan: Brief (longer in mosaic Trisomy 13)

*Edwards Syndrome* (Chromosome 18)

- Rare
- Neurologic features: Severe intellectual disability, seizures, hypotonia, microcephaly
- Non-neurologic features: Camptodactyly, heart defects
- Typical lifespan: Brief (longer in mosaic Trisomy 18)

*Down Syndrome* (Trisomy of Chromosome 21)

- About 1 in 700 live births
- Neurologic features: Variable intellectual disability, hypotonia, seizures
- Non-neurologic features: Endocardial cushion defects, short fingers/toes
- Increased Alzheimer's disease risk: Gene for amyloid precursor protein is on Chromosome 21
- Acute lymphoblastic leukemia (ALL) is common in Down syndrome
- Typical lifespan: Highly variable

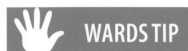

**WARDS TIP**

Some people believe Fragile X only affects male children but female children can also be affected, though the presentation is typically more mild.

**WARDS TIP**

Feel like an angel: Happy and laughing.

**WARDS TIP**

On the wards, Angelman and Prader-Willi are always discussed together as the best described example of genetic "imprinting," the phenomenon in which different phenotypes are seen when the pathologic mutation is inherited from the mother or the father. Practically, these conditions have little to do with each other and are rarely on the differential in the same patient. Prader-Willi is typically diagnosed in neonates with hypotonia and feeding problems, whereas Angelman is usually diagnosed in infants with seizures and developmental concerns.

## DEVELOPMENTAL DELAY SYNDROMES

### Fragile X

- Genetic mutation of FMR1 (encoding FMRP) on Chromosome X.
- Incidence about 1 in 7000 and often called the most commonly identified genetic cause of autism/intellectual disability.
- Think big/long symptoms: Long, narrow face, large ears, prominent jaw, macroorchidism.
- Early intervention developmental services are the best-known treatments.

### Rett Syndrome

- Genetic mutation of MECP2 on Chromosome X.
- Incidence 1 in 10,000.
- Characteristic history involves initial normal development followed by marked *developmental regression* (losing milestones previously gained) with flattening of head circumference growth.
  - Many children developed repetitive hand movements most characteristically described as holding their hands together in the middle of the body and "wringing" them.
  - Seizures are common.
  - Many children develop a characteristic pattern of apnea/breath-holding.
  - Many children require G-Tubes but often have severe retching.

### Angelman Syndrome

- Rare mutation of Chromosome 15 on a maternally inherited copy, most typically the *Ube3A* gene. Typical presentation is developmental delay, sleep problems, and seizures with a characteristic EEG finding (notched delta waves) in infants.
- Definitive test is a "methylation assay" in which the pattern by which methyl groups are arrayed on the gene are inspected to determine if the mutated gene is maternal or paternal in origin.

### Prader-Willi Syndrome (PWS)

- Rare mutation of Chromosome 15 on a paternally inherited copy, possibly involving the UBE3A region.
- Definitive test: Methylation assay.
- Typical presentation: Hypotonia and poor feeding in a neonate.
  - When older, children with PWS often develop voracious appetites and will eat until extremely obese. Some lash out violently if denied food.
- Treatment: Calorie restriction and hormone substitution.

**Case 1:** An 8-year-old child with rapid downward deviation of both eyes followed by slow upward conjugate eye movements probably has which of the following?

A.  SSPE
B.  MS
C.  Pontine glioma
D.  Cervicomedullary junction ischemia

The correct answer is C. Lesions of the pons can give rise to "ocular bobbing" which is described in this case.

**Case 2:** A 9-year-old girl has large port-wine spots on her right forehead, contralateral (left-sided) hemiparesis, intellectual disability, and seizures, as well as glaucoma. Skull radiographs reveal intracranial calcifications that are associated with leptomeningeal angiomatosis. What is the diagnosis?

A.  Sturge-Weber syndrome
B.  Von Hippel-Lindau syndrome
C.  Edwards syndrome
D.  Down syndrome
E.  Lennox-Gastaut syndrome

The correct answer is A. This patient has classic findings of Sturge-Weber syndrome.

**Case 3:** A 23-year-old female patient with bilateral acoustic neuromas also has café-au-lait spots on her back and legs. She also has a family history of bilateral hearing loss at a relatively young age. A gene abnormality should be suspected on which chromosome?

A.  4
B.  9
C.  17
D.  21
E.  22

The correct answer is E. Meningiomas and bilateral acoustic neuromas occur in type 2 neurofibromatosis, a dominantly inherited disorder arising with a gene deletion on Chr 22. NF1 is associated with chromosome 17. People with NF1 are commonly affected by cutaneous manifestations, but would not be expected to have a family history of bilateral hearing loss at a young age.

## NOTES

# CHAPTER 14

# SLEEP DISORDERS

In this chapter, we will review sleep disorders that can involve difficulties related to sleeping, including difficulty falling or staying asleep or, falling asleep at inappropriate times, excessive sleep, or abnormal behaviors associated with sleep.

## Insomnia

- Difficulty with sleep initiation, maintenance, and duration, or subjective quality
- Can be primary (psychophysiological or behavioral) or secondary (med effect)

## Sleep-Related Breathing Disorders

- Obstructive sleep apnea vs central sleep apnea
  - Criteria for OSA: daytime sleepiness, loud snoring, witnessed breathing interruptions, or awakenings due to gasping/choking AND at least five obstructive respiratory events
    - Obstructive respiratory events: apnea, hypopnea, respiratory effort-related awakenings
  - Central apnea causes: Cheyne stokes (crescendo-decrescendo pattern of tidal volumes followed by a period of apnea) and primary sleep apnea of infancy (prematurity)
- Treatment:
  - Weight loss
  - Continuous positive airway pressure (CPAP)
  - Tonsillectomy in children
  - Mandibular surgery

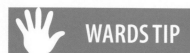

**WARDS TIP**

3 Cs of central sleep apnea—Congestive heart failure, CNS toxicity or trauma, Cheyne-Stokes breathing

## Hypersomnias

Daytime sleepiness not due to disturbed nocturnal sleep.

### NARCOLEPSY (WITH OR WITHOUT CATAPLEXY)

- Symptoms: Excessive daytime somnolence ≥3 months, sleep attacks, cataplexy (pathognomonic, abrupt onset of REM atonia triggered by strong emotional stimuli or physical exercise) varying severity, weakness most frequent at the knee, sleep paralysis.
- May experience hypnagogic (just before sleep) or hypnopompic (just before awakening) hallucination.
- Onset at any age—usually second decade of life.
- Diagnosis: Overnight polysomnogram and multiple sleep latency test.

- Etiology:
  - Hypocretin (orexin) deficiency leads to narcolepsy with cataplexy.
  - Treatment:
    - Modafinil first line.
    - Daily naps and avoidance of sleep deprivation.
    - Stimulants (eg, methylphenidate, amphetamines).
    - TCAs (eg, clomipramine) for cataplexy.

## SLEEP-ASSOCIATED MOVEMENT DISORDERS

- Restless leg syndrome (RLS):
  - Autosomal-dominant inheritance pattern.
  - Most commonly idiopathic but sometimes secondary to some chronic conditions (eg, iron deficiency, ESRD), drugs (eg, lithium, antidepressants), and pregnancy.
  - Treatment:
    - Iron supplementation.
    - Discontinue offending drugs.
    - Consider dopamine agonists and anticonvulsants (eg, gabapentin).

## PERIODIC LIMB MOVEMENT DISORDER (PLMD—FORMERLY CALLED SLEEP MYOCLONUS OR NOCTURNAL MYOCLONUS)

- Described as repetitive limb movements that occur during sleep and cause sleep disruption.
- Usually involves the lower extremities, consisting of extension of the big toe and flexion of the ankle, the knee, and the hip.
- Limb movements can occur in the upper extremities as well.
- Observed in about 80% of patients with RLS.
- PLMS can occur in over 30% of people aged 65 and older and can be asymptomatic.
- Common in patients with narcolepsy and REM behavior disorder, and may be seen in patients with obstructive sleep apnea.
- The limb movements occur most frequently in light non-REM sleep.
- Dopamine agonists are considered first line of treatment.

## Parasomnias

Undesirable phenomena that occur while falling asleep, during sleep, and while waking (Table 14-1).

**TABLE 14-1. The Various Types of Parasomnias**

| | Sleep Terror | Nightmare | Confusional Arousal | Sleepwalking/Somnambulism | REM Sleep Behavior Disorder | Nocturnal Seizure | Rhythmic Movement Disorder | Hypnic Jerks |
|---|---|---|---|---|---|---|---|---|
| **Behavior** | Autonomic arousal, screaming, motor activity | Less intense vocalization, fear, motor activity | Confused; semipurposeful, complex behavior with eyes open | Complex behaviors not limited to walking | Acting out dreams, sometimes combative, may be violent | Variable, but stereotyped | Head banging or body rocking that occurs prior to or in light sleep | Brief movement, sound, or sensation at sleep onset |
| **Age of onset** | Childhood | Any age | Childhood/adolescence | Any age; peak incidence in early adolescence | Older adult (may herald a neurodegenerative disorder such as Parkinson disease or Lewy body dementia) | Anytime | Early childhood | Any age |
| **Time of occurrence** | First 90 minutes of sleep | Second half of night | First third of night | First third of night | Last third of night | Anytime | Prior to sleep onset | Sleep onset |
| **Duration** | Usually <3 minutes | <30 minutes | Minutes | Variable; can be long | Seconds to minutes | <3 minutes | Minutes to hours | <1 second |
| **Memory of event** | No | Yes | No | No | Dream recall | No | Yes | Yes |
| **Polysomnogram finding** | Slow-wave sleep | REM | Slow-wave sleep | Slow-wave sleep | REM sleep but with ↑ EMG tone | Potentially epileptiform activity | Light sleep | Brief ↓ in EMG prior to myoclonus |
| **Treatment** | Behavioral | Behavioral | Benzodiazepines | Benzodiazepines; tricyclics | Clonazepam, carbamazepine | Antiepileptic drug | Behavioral | Behavioral |

**Case 1:** A 6-year-old boy has had recurrent night-time episodes of screaming, intense fear, and flailing while still asleep. His mother describes him as sitting up in bed and appearing frightened. He has a wide-eyed stare and appears to be perspiring, breathing heavily, and have a racing pulse. The episode lasts 5 to 10 minutes and usually occurs soon after falling asleep. He is hard to awaken and has no memory of the event the next morning. What is his diagnosis?

A. Nightmare
B. Sleep terror
C. Confusional arousal
D. Medication reaction

The correct answer is B. The symptoms are most consistent with Sleep Terrors which occur soon after falling asleep, with no recollection of the behavioral episode which consists of screaming and thrashing about.

**Case 2:** A 29-year-old male describes a strange inability to move while awakening in the morning. He says it can last 5 to 10 minutes in duration. He also describes visual hallucinations when falling asleep at night. He notes that sometimes at work he experiences vivid dreams while he is awake. He describes a feeling of levitation and reports chronic excessive daytime sleepiness with sleep attacks. He denies any drug abuse and no seizure history. What is the diagnosis?

A. Parkinsonism
B. Narcolepsy with Cataplexy
C. Narcolepsy without Cataplexy
D. Vestibular migraine
E. Hysteria

The correct answer is B. This patient has the classic constellation of Narcolepsy with Cataplexy, including hypnogogic hallucinations and sleep paralysis. The sense of levitation is the Cenesthopathy syndrome which can be associated with narcolepsy.

**Case 3:** An obese 45-year-old male with type 2 diabetes, hypertension, and hyperlipidemia presents with his wife for a chief complaint of "snoring so loud the house shakes." He is also noticing difficulty working in the afternoons when he develops significant sleepiness, so much so that he needs to take a 30- to 45-minute nap. His wife states that his snoring has become worse in the past year and she has started to sleep at her sister's house down the street. What is the best treatment for his condition?

A. Weight loss
B. Continuous positive airway pressure (CPAP)
C. A and B
D. High doses of caffeine
E. Modafinil

The correct answer is C. The combination of weight loss and CPAP should help improve this patient's (and his wife's) situation where effects of sleep apnea and its associated snoring can be mitigated with weight loss and CPAP.

**NOTES**

# INDEX

Page numbers followed by "f" denote figures; those followed by "t" denote tables.